Pain and its Origins, Diagnosis and Treatments

Nerve Growth Factor and Pain

PAIN AND ITS ORIGINS, DIAGNOSIS AND TREATMENTS

Acute Pain: Causes, Effects and Treatment
Sam D'Alonso and Katherine L. Grasso (Editors)
2009. ISBN: 978-1-67041-223-6

Nerve Growth Factor and Pain
Paola Sarchielli, Katiuscia Nardi, Stefano Caproni, Davide Chiasserini, Alessio Pieroni, Ilenia Corbelli and Paolo Calabresi
2010. ISBN: 978-1-61668-264-4

Nerve Growth Factor and Pain
Paola Sarchielli, Katiuscia Nardi, Stefano Caproni, Davide Chiasserini, Alessio Pieroni, Ilenia Corbelli and Paolo Calabresi
2010. ISBN: 978-1-61668-698-7 (E-book)

Pain and its Origins, Diagnosis and Treatments

NERVE GROWTH FACTOR AND PAIN

PAOLA SARCHIELLI, KATIUSCIA NARDI,
STEFANO CAPRONI, DAVIDE CHIASSERINI,
ALESSIO PIERONI, ILENIA CORBELLI
AND PAOLO CALABRESI

Nova Science Publishers, Inc.
New York

LIBRARY OF CONGRESS CATALOGING-IN-PUBLICATION DATA

Available upon Request
ISBN: 978-1-61668-264-4

Published by Nova Science Publishers, Inc. † New York

CONTENTS

PREFACE

Nerve growth factor (NGF) has a key role not only in the development of sensory and autonomic neurons, but also in the processes of nociception. Several central and peripheral mechanisms have been postulated as the basis of effects of NGF in nociceptive pathways. It has been implicated both in inflammatory and neuropathic pain mechanisms and strategies against NGF, its receptors, belonging to the tyrosine kinase (Trk) family, and down-stream intracellular signaling activated by this neurotrophin (NT) have been proposed for the treatment of these pathological conditions.

There is also recent evidence of the involvement of NGF in other painful diseases, such as migraine, in particular in the chronic form, and fibromyalgia. This suggests the potential usefulness of anti-NGF strategies as novel analgesics also for these disabling pathological conditions.

Paola Sarchielli[1*], Katiuscia Nardi[1], Stefano Caproni[1], Davide Chiasserini[1], Alessio Pieroni[1], Ilenia Corbelli[1] and Paolo Calabresi[1,2]

[1] Neurologic Clinic, Department of Medical and Surgical Specialities and Public Health, University of Perugia, Italy

[2] IRCCS, Santa Lucia Foundation, European Brain Research Institute, Rome, Italy

[*] Corresponding author: Dr. Paola Sarchielli, Neurologic Clinic, Department of Medical and Surgical Specialties and Public Health, University of Perugia, Ospedale Santa Maria della Misericordia, Località Sant'Andrea delle Fratte, San Sisto, 06158 Perugia, Italy, Tel.: +39 075 578 3562; Fax: +39 075 578 4229, E-mail addresses: paola.sarchielli@gmail.com

INTRODUCTION

Nerve growth factor (NGF) was the first neurotrophin (NT) to be identified, and its role in the development and survival of both peripheral and central sensory neurons has been well characterized [Wiesmann et al, 2001]. Among its effects in the post-natal period, a great deal of attention has focused on the involvement of NGF in pain mechanisms [Nicol et al, 2007].

NGF is produced by a number of cell types including keratinocytes [Di Marco et al, 1993], mast cells [Leon et al., 1994], B-lymphocytes [Torcia et al, 1996], fibroblasts [Lindholm et al, 1990], bronchial epithelial cells [Kassel et al, 2001], renal mesangial cells [Steiner et al, 1991], smooth muscle cells [Ueyama et al, 1993], and skeletal muscle myotubes [Schwartz et al, 2002]. This NT up-regulates the expression of sensory neuropeptides in nociceptive neurons, and its activity is mediated through two different membrane-bound receptors, the tyrosine kinase A (TrkA) receptor and the p75 receptor [Pezet & McMahon, 2006]. The latter receptor is structurally related to other members of the tumor necrosis factor (TNF) receptor family, which have been found on a variety of cell types also outside of the nervous system [Pezet & McMahon, 2006].

NGF appears to act by multiple mechanisms which include: i) changes in the peripheral and central sensory neurons including nociceptive neurons; ii) changes in the expression of genes responsible for nerve activation and conduction such as ion channels and some pain-related receptors; iii) axonal growth and nerve degeneration; iv) induction of brain-derived neurotrophic factor (BDNF), which, in turn, intervenes in pain signal processing within the spinal cord [Pezet & McMahon, 2006].

The above evidence supports, therefore, the central role of NGF in nociception, in particular, in inflammatory pain or neuropathic pain. In addition, elevated levels of NGF have been detected in tissues, cerebrospinal fluid (CSF), and central venous blood in a number of painful diseases, such as visceral pain, post-surgical pain, fibromyalgia and also migraine, in particular, in chronic migraine [Giovengo et al, 1999; Sarchielli et al, 2001; Sarchielli et al, 2002; Sarchielli et al, 2007b]. The ability of this NT to increase nociception had raised the idea that compounds targeting NGF, its TrkA receptor and down-stream intracellular signaling would be a promising alternative treatment for acute and chronic intractable pain [Sarchielli et al, 2004a]. Their administration has been proposed for potentiation of the effects of opioid analgesics on severe pain, with consequent reduction of dosage and undesirable side effects [Cahill et al, 2003]. In alternative, antagonistic compounds of NGF were also considered for mild-moderate pain or for the preventive treatment of various chronic painful diseases [Owolabi et al, 1999].

The present review highlights the role of NGF in nociception during adulthood and, beginning with experimental and clinical evidence, illustrates the most relevant knowledge concerning the pathogenic mechanisms of inflammatory and neuropathic pain, as well as migraine and fibromyalgia, with particular regard to the involvement of NGF. Finally, it provides the most recent findings on the potential role of therapeutic strategies targeting NGF in inflammatory and neuropathic pain and, potentially, in migraine and fibromyalgia.

Chapter 1

NGF AND NOCICEPTION

NGF has been clearly shown to be involved in the embryonic development of sensory neurons, including nociceptive sensory neurons [Ritter et al, 1991]. In addition, an altered expression of this NT factor and its receptors contributes to plastic changes in primary afferents during the early neonatal period consequent to peripheral inflammatory events [Chien et al, 2007].

Nociceptive neurons require this NT to maintain their phenotype also in the post-natal period. Moreover, TrkA receptors continue to be expressed in these neurons, which synthesize this NT also after embryonic development [Mendell et al, 1999]. Even in adulthood, NGF regulates specification of the nociceptive phenotype [Koltzenburg, 1999; Bennett, 2001].

Experimental evidence showed that NGF is released by several cell types, including mast cells [Bienenstock et al, 1987; Skaper et al, 2001], monocytes/macrophages [Bracci-Laudiero et al, 2005], lymphocytes [Bonini et al, 2003] and also Schwann cells [Créange, 1997] in response to tissue inflammation. In addition, an increase in NGF production can be triggered by a variety of stimuli, which include proinflammatory cytokines, such as interleukin (IL)-1β, tumor necrosis factor (TNF-α), IL-4 and platelet-derived growth factor (PDGF) produced by inflammatory cells [Levi-Montalcini et al, 1996; Woolf et al, 1997].

NGF is responsible for hyperalgesia when administered locally, systemically or intrathecally in different animal species [Brodie, 1995; Hao et al, 2000]. This hyperalgesic effect of NGF emerged both from experiments investigating behavioral responses in humans and from pain perception models in animals and humans [Pezet & McMahon, 2006; Della Seta et al, 1994;

Amann et al, 1995]. In animal models NGF-induced thermal hyperalgesia occurs within an hour after its administration. Both this short latency and the local effect of NGF support the involvement of a prevalent peripheral mechanism [Shu & Mendell, 1999]. NGF-induced mechanical hyperalgesia develops, in contrast, with a latency of some hours, suggesting the activation of more complex central mechanisms [Ma & Woolf, 1997; Hathway et al, 2006].

Pain-related behavioral responses to NGF in animals also manifest within minutes but last hours or days, depending on the dose and route of administration [Zahn et al, 2004; Lewin et al, 1994]. Similar effects have been shown in human volunteers in whom administration of small amounts of NGF, subcutaneously or intramuscularly, induces pain and tenderness at the site of injection, which start within minutes and persist for several hours. Likewise, small intravenous NGF doses are responsible for widespread deep pain and tenderness that may persist for several days [Svensson et al, 2003].

Chapter 2

INTRACELLULAR MECHANISMS OF NGF ACTION

The role played by NGF in peripheral nociception is emphasized by the evidence of the up-regulation and increased delivery of this NT and over-expression of high-affinity TrkA receptors in the nociceptive terminals in the injured areas after inflammatory insults [Pezet et al, 1999]. The hyperalgesic action of NGF in inflammatory pain models may, in part, be the consequence of the increased sensitivity of peripheral nociceptive terminals. This increased sensitivity is due to a direct action of NGF on TrkA-expressing Aδ ad C fibers via the enhancement of the release of substance P (SP), calcitonin gene-related peptide (CGRP), and other sensitizing mediators from TrkA-expressing cells, post-ganglion sympathetic neurons, mast cells and immune cells in the site of inflammatory insult or after peripheral NGF administration [Woolf et al, 1996; Malcangio et al, 1997, 2000].

TrkA activation, after interaction with NGF, leads to the induction of several intracellular signaling cascades affecting the sensitivity of nociceptive afferents. The retrograde signal mediated by the internalized TrkA-NGF complex transported in sensory neurons to the dorsal root ganglion (DRG) alters the transcription of several proteins and peptides [Wehrman et al, 2007]. Genes differentially expressed include, in particular, sensory neuropeptides, receptors and voltage-regulated ion channels [Chao et al, 2006; Malik-Hall et al, 2005; Molliver et al, 2005].

In particular, the exogenous NGF administration *in vivo* or the addition of NGF *in vitro* to cultured sensory neurons induces the increase in messenger RNA (mRNA) and protein levels of both neuropeptides SP and CGRP in cell bodies [Vedder et al, 1993]. The remodeling of CGRP fibers surrounding

NGF-immunoreactive cell bodies, the increase in CGRP and SP as well as the over-expression of neurokinin K1 (NK1) receptor due to NGF is a slow process, requiring from hours to days to manifest itself. These modifications confirm, therefore, the implication of transcriptional mechanisms, which may account for a long-lasting sensitization that contributes to the maintenance of painful sensation [McMahon, 1996].

A number of ligand-gated ion channels, normally expressed throughout the sensory neurons and concentrated at both peripheral and central axonal arbors, are also regulated by NGF in neurons bearing TrkA receptors. They include transient receptor potential vanilloid 1 ($TRPV_1$), acid-sensing ion channels (ASIC3), purinergic receptors of adenosine triphosphate (ATP) 2X3 (P2X3), G protein–coupled receptors, such as bradykinin (BK) B_2 receptors, and the μ opiate receptors [Xue et al, 2007; Amaya et al, 2004; Mamet et al, 2003; Ramer et al, 2001; Lee et al, 2002]. Specifically, sensitization of nociceptive afferents seems to be related to the enhanced responsiveness of $TRPV_1$ receptor due to its phosphorylation [Cortright & Szallasi, 2004]. The intracellular cascades related to $TRPV_1$ sensitization have not been completely clarified, but phosphatidylinositol 3-kinase (PI3K) and the mitogen-activated protein kinase (MAPK)/extracellular signal-regulated kinase (ERK) pathways seem to be the most likely candidates [Zhang et al, 2005; Zhuang et al, 2004; Zhu & Oxford, 2007].

A further effect of NGF is the regulation of the voltage-gated ion channels genes, which include calcium (Ca^{2+}), potassium (K^+) and Na^+ channels [Pezet & McMahon, 2006]. In particular, both tetrodotoxin-resistant (TTX-r) and tetrodotoxin-sensitive (TTX-s) Na^+ currents are increased in DRG neurons by NGF [Woodall et al, 2007; Park et al, 2003; Okuse et al, 1997]. Multiple α subunits, including Nav 1.3, 1.7, 1.8, and 1.9 are regulated by NGF, and this effect of endogenously produced or exogenously administered NGF has functional consequences on the sensory transduction/transmission of nociceptive information [Gould et al, 2000; Leffler, 2002; Fjell et al, 1999; Kerr et al, 2001; Amaya et al, 2006].

Through the above mechanism, NGF-induced changes have, therefore, a great impact on the excitability of nociceptive neuron excitability, as shown by increased spontaneous activity registered in DRG neurons in the presence of NGF [Djouhri et al, 2001; Kitamura et al, 2005].

A further pivotal effect of NGF is the upregulation of BDNF in DRG and the central afferents of nociceptive neurons [Michael et al, 1997]. This NT, which is normally expressed in approximately 30-40% of DRG neurons [Apfel et al, 1996] and trigeminal neurons [Ichikawa et al, 2006], is induced in virtually all TrkA-expressing neurons after NGF treatment [Michael et al, 1997].

Chapter 3

Pathophysiological Mechanisms of Inflammatory and Neuropathic Pain

Available information obtained from experimental animal models suggests that both inflammatory and neuropathic pain result from cellular and neuroplastic changes occurring in both the peripheral and central nervous system (CNS). A series of processes have been observed that, singly or in combination, may explain the symptoms pointed out in individual patients [Scholz & Woolf, 2002]. In the periphery, following tissue damage or an event that causes direct nerve damage, an inflammatory response ensues. Both inflammatory cells and peripheral neurons in the site of nerve insult release various chemical mediators, including 5-hydroxytryptamine (5-HT), BK, SP, CGRP, histamine, ATP, proinflammatory cytokines, and products from the cyclooxygenase and lipoxygenase pathways of arachidonic acid metabolism. The above substances induce the activation of peripheral nociceptive afferents, and the severity of nociceptive pain is correlated with the extent of tissue damage, and if tissue healing occurs, pain tends to lessen or disappear [Sutherland et al, 2000].

Conversely, neuropathic pain may be initiated by a relatively modest physical insult, and the severity of neuropathic pain does not always correlate with the extent of neuronal damage. As a consequence, significant negative neurologic symptoms such as sensory deficit, weakness and reflex changes, indicative of significant nerve injury, can be, in some cases, prevalent with scarce or no pain. In other cases, acute pain can occur and be the prevailing symptom. In addition, there may be paresthesias, dysesthesias (abnormal or unpleasant sensations without true pain), or spontaneous pain [Bowsher & Haggett, 2005]. In both conditions of inflammatory and neuropathic pain, sensitization of peripheral nociceptive afferents results in an increased responsiveness to thermal and mechanical stimuli, which is mediated through thin, unmyelinated C-fiber primary afferent neurons. This is the most accepted hypothesis regarding the mechanism of hyperalgesia [Siddall & Cousins, 1997; Woolf & Chong, 1993]. If demyelination of the nerve occurs (e.g., Aβ or Aδ fibers), ectopic discharges along the length of the nerve fiber may provide sustained afferent input to the spinal cord. These ectopic signals may persist for extended periods of time and are believed to play a role in the initiation and maintenance of neuropathic pain. Continuous discharge in C fibers may produce sensations of burning pain, whereas intermittent spontaneous discharge in Aβ or Aδ fibers is responsible for lancinating dysesthesias or paresthesias [Petersen & Rowbotham, 2000]. In addition, a neuroma may form at the site of injury, which is responsible not only for spontaneous pain, but also for hyperalgesia and paresthesias [Wall & Gutnick, 1974; Govrin-Lippmann & Devor, 1978].

Neuropathic pain syndromes may be divided into two groups, central and peripheral, based on the location of the nervous system lesion. Following nerve damage, the neuropathic mechanisms can expand during the disease and lead to both peripheral and central pathological changes, making the distinction between peripheral and central pain less distinct than once believed. An example is post-herpetic neuralgia (PHN), which is a persistent pain in the area of a herpes zoster outbreak. PHN involves damage to the peripheral nervous system (DRG), but this can result in anatomic changes in the DH in the CNS, thus making PHN a neuropathic pain with mixed central and peripheral components [Oaklander, 2008].

Changes in the expression of ion channels and receptors have been observed in peripheral and spinal cord afferent pathway underlying inflammatory and neuropathic pain. Specifically, an alteration in voltage-dependent Na^+ and Ca^{2+} channel subunits has been shown after chronic nerve injury associated with neuropathic pain [Matzner & Devor, 1994]. These include an increase in the expression of Nav1.3 channels and Na^+ channel β3 (Navβ3), Ca^{2+} channel α2αδ1 (Cavα2δ-1) subunits in DRG neuron cell bodies, and in the expression of Nav1.3 in second-order nociceptive neurons in the spinal cord dorsal horn (DH) of the spinal cord [Cummins et al, 2001]. The TTX-r Na^+ channel subunits Nav1.8 and Nav1.9 are also redistributed from DRG neuron cell bodies to peripheral axons and pain receptors at the site of injury [Cummins & Waxman, 1997]. Nav 1.9, in particular, is the more relevant effector of the hypersensitivity produced by multiple inflammatory mediators on nociceptive peripheral terminals [Amaya et al, 2006]. A role for the TTX-r Na^+ channel Nav 1.8 in NGF-induced hyperalgesia has also been demonstrated [Kerr et al, 2001].

Abnormal ectopic discharges from neuromas also seem to be caused by alterations in the expression of the different Na^+ ion channel subtypes that are involved in lowering the threshold for mechanical activation [Ro & Chang, 2005]. Furthermore, a pivotal role emerged for TRP channels, a family of evolutionarily conserved ligand-gated ion channels. Six TRPs ($TRPV_1$, $TRPV_2$, $TRPV_3$, $TRPV_4$, $TRPM_8$ and TRPA1) are expressed in primary nociceptive neurons, where they act as transducers for thermal, chemical and mechanical stimuli. They have been demonstrated to contribute to pain hypersensitivity associated with peripheral inflammatory and neuropathic pain states [Levine & Alessandri-Haber, 2007]. Among these receptors, in particular, the nociceptor-specific ion channel $TRPV_1$ serves as the molecular target of capsaicin. It can also be activated by noxious heat (with a thermal threshold >43° C) or low pH and endogenous lipids, and all these stimuli are known to cause pain *in vivo* [Palazzo et al, 2008]. Furthermore, studies using $TRPV_1$-deficient mice have shown that $TRPV_1$ is essential for selective modalities of pain sensation and thermal hyperalgesia [Roberts & Connor, 2006].

Sensitization of $TRPV_1$ is one mechanism that has been recognized to initiate pain by tissue damage/inflammation [Huang et al, 2006]. Phenotypic change of primary afferents with respect to expression of $TRPV_1$ channels may also account for some paroxysmal symptoms and signs in neuropathic pain [Katsura et al, 2006]. $TRPV_1$ receptors are expressed in the CNS, where they seem to play a pivotal role in pain mediated by central sensitization. They can also be the target of specific agonists, whose penetration into the CNS is essential for producing a broad-spectrum analgesia [Cui et al, 2006]. However, if the $TRPV_1$ receptor plays a pro-nociceptive role in certain models of acute tissue injury, under chronic polyneuropathic conditions it can initiate anti-nociceptive counter-regulatory mechanisms possibly mediated by somatostatin released from sensory neurons [Helyes et al, 2007].

In addition to $TRPV_1$, the other five thermosensitive ion channels in mammals, $TRPV_2$, $TRPV_3$, $TRPV_4$, $TRPM_8$ and $TRPA_1$ act within the noxious range of temperatures and may further contribute to pain due to inflammatory injury [Numazaki & Tominaga, 2004; Bölcskei et al, 2003].

Further molecular sensors detecting adverse stimuli can be activated by inflammatory signals, causing primary hyperalgesia [Coutaux et al., 2005]. Among them, the PX receptor channels, the molecular sensor for ATP, are implicated in hyperalgesia accompanying tissue damage [Donnelly-Roberts et al, 2008]. Their expression is increased in animal models of neuropathic pain [Chen et al, 2005]. Moreover, the specific 5-HT receptor subtype expressed in nociceptive endings, 5-HT_{3R}, seems to be involved in the activation of nociceptive neurons by 5-HT released from activated platelets and enterochromaffin cells [Meuser et al, 2002].

The increased susceptibility to firing and the increased firing frequency of sensitized peripheral nociceptive afferents are responsible for the so-called phenomenon of "central sensitization" that refers to neuroplastic changes involving second-order nociceptive neurons, which is believed to account for the clinical phenomenon of allodynia [Garcia-Larrea & Magnin, 2008].

Plastic changes of the DH neurons is implicated in the increase in receptive field size, the increase in the magnitude and duration of the response to stimuli, and the reduction in their excitatory threshold. Under these conditions, central neurons that normally receive high-threshold sensory input may begin to receive input from low-threshold mechanoreceptors. This information may be interpreted as nociceptive [Katz & Rothenberg, 2005].

An alternative hypothesis is that allodynia is caused by a decrease in central inhibition of the mechanically-induced nociceptive input. Furthermore, within the spinal cord, collateral sprouting of primary afferent neurons may occur [Garcia-Larrea & Magnin, 2008]. Accordingly, nerve fibers in deeper laminae that do not normally transmit pain sprout into more superficial regions of the DH (e.g., laminae I and II) and become receptive to nociceptive input. Another possible mechanism for central sensitization is ephaptic conduction, also known as "crosstalk" between neurons [Soderling & Derkach, 2000]. Chemical mediators lower, in fact, the threshold for cross-excitation, which becomes sufficient to evoke ectopic firing from a biochemical and molecular point of view. Experimental findings suggest that central sensitization is mediated through the release of various neurotransmitters [e.g., SP, glutamate, CGRP, γ-aminobutyric acid (GABA), and NKA, production of nitric oxide (NO) by NO synthase and through activation of the N-methyl-D-aspartate (NMDA) receptor, increased Ca^{2+} flux (possibly through N-type calcium channels], and prostaglandin synthesis [Petrenko et al, 2003; Omoigui, 2007].

In the last few years, the intervention of some NTs in persisting pain states has been emphasized. In particular, NGF has been demonstrated to play a pivotal role in diffuse inflammatory and neuropathic pain conditions by regulating sensory neuron phenotype and excitability.

Chapter 4

Experimental Evidence for the Involvement of NGF in Inflammatory and Neuropathic Pain

The increase of both NGF mRNA and protein has been demonstrated in different experimental models of inflammatory pain, where this NT acts as an algogenic mediator produced by skin keratocytes, Schwann cells, macrophages, mast cells and T cells. Examples of inflammatory conditions in experimental animals, in which NGF has been implicated, include models of cutaneous carragenin, lipopolysaccharide (LPS), complete Freund's adjuvant (CFA), skin wounds, muscle formalin, acute injury, arthritis, spinal cord injury disc herniation, acute burn injury, bone cancer-pain, acute pancreatitis and incisional pain [Kanaan et al, 1998; Safieh-Garabedian et al, 2002; Talhouk et al, 2004; Woolf et al, 1997; Djouhri et al, 2001; Cruise et al, 2004; Ueda et al, 2002; Krenz &Weaver, 2000; Obata et al, 2004a; Toma et al, 2000; Saban et al, 2002; Wu et al, 2007; Zahn et al, 2004].

In contrast, in several neuropathic conditions characterized by sensory loss, peripheral nerve injury leads to a down-regulation of NGF, which is responsible for some changes occurring in TrkA-expressing neurons, typically over several days or weeks. This has been demonstrated in the case of axotomy and includes a down-regulation of the neuropeptides SP and CGRP and, conversely, an up-regulation of galanin, vasoactive intestinal peptide, and activating transcription factor 3. The above changes can be prevented by a few micrograms of NGF delivered via an osmotic pump onto the end of the sciatic nerve [Fitzgerald et al, 1985] or intrathecally [Verge et al, 1992]. Similarly, a down-regulation of $TRPV_1$, Nav 1.8 and Nav 1.9 is induced by axotomy, and is reversed by NGF [Gould et al, 2000]. Other transmitters and receptors in non-TrkA neurons, (mainly large mechanosensitive cells and small non peptidergic neurons), constitutively expressing the P2X3 receptor, are unaffected by NGF treatment [Averill et al, 2004]. NGF also protects damaged sensory neurons from high doses of capsaicin, which is recognized to induce a loss of axon terminals and a decrease of sensory neuropeptide expression [Donnerer et al, 2005]

A neuroprotective effect of NGF was also demonstrated following damage to the central branch of the primary sensory neurons, such as in the case of dorsal root avulsion [Romero et al, 2001]. They undergo wallerian degeneration and DH neurons lose their afferent input. Injured sensory neurons can regenerate within the DH and this phenomenon is dependent on NGF availability [Romero et al, 2001].

Further recent evidence suggests that regeneration of the peripheral branches of sensory neurons and neurite outgrowth of subpopulations of injured sensory neurons due to NGF occur, as with NT-3. This seems to be mediated by α-7 integrin and laminin signaling [Gardiner et al, 2005]. NGF also restores the *in vivo* expression of voltage gated Na^+ channels, which is reduced in the case of peripheral nerve damage in some neuropathic models in rats, such as the L5/6 thigh nerve ligation or axotomy [Okuse et al, 1997].

Furthermore, experimental findings support a role for NGF in preventing semaphorin 3A-mediated growth cone collapse in adult neurons, in which this chemorepellent guides centrally projecting axons of DRG. A similar effect is shared by glial cell line-derived neurotrophic factor (GDNF), neurturin or cyclic adenosine 5'-monophosphate (cAMP). This novel converging signaling pathway could possibly be used as a therapeutic option for neuropathic pain, and needs to be explored in future research [Wanigasekara & Keast, 2006].

In contrast, recent data suggest that the NGF precursor (pro-NGF) may function as a death-inducing ligand mediating its apoptotic effects via p75NTR. Pro-NGF-induced apoptosis seems to be dependent upon membrane expression of the sortilin receptor, which interacts with p75NTR to promote a high-affinity binding site for pro-NGF, as demonstrated in the model of sciatic nerve transection. The relevance of this finding for sensory neuron loss needs to be established in experimental neuropathic models [Arnett et al, 2007].

NGF dramatically upregulates pituitary adenylate cyclase-activating polypeptide (PACAP) expression in TrkA-positive neurons in both intact and injured DRGs in the model of chronic constriction injury (CCI). Also, galanin expression in adult sensory neurons was modulated by NGF in injured neurons and after inflammatory insult. The elevated expression of both PACAP and galanin in injured neurons is mitigated by NT-3, suggesting a role for this NT, but not NGF, in returning the 'injured phenotype' back towards an 'intact phenotype' without modifying TrkA mRNA expression due to CCI of the sciatic nerve [Wilson-Gerwing & Verge, 2006].

Diabetic neuropathy is a prototypic condition in which peripheral sensory nerves are compromised in their ability to transport NTs, mainly NGF [Apfel, 1999], and in which a reduction of $TRPV_1$ levels has been observed as a result of NGF decrease [Facer et al, 2007; Anand et al, 2006]. The depletion of NGF in human diabetic neuropathy skin has been correlated with the dysfunctioning of nociceptive fibers [Anand, 2004]. Similar mechanisms can be hypothesized even for Human Immunodeficiency Virus (HIV) neuropathy.

The above observations prompted the design of NGF administration trials involving both diabetic and HIV patients, which failed, however, to show any significant effect on antagonizing the sensory alterations in patient outcome [McArthur et al, 2000; Larkin, 1998; Schifitto et al, 2001], perhaps because of the difficulty in identifying appropriate doses and the probable need for multiple trophic factors, in contrast to the beneficial effects observed in animal models [Apfel, 2002; Christianson et al, 2007].

In experimental models of diabetic neuropathy, the majority of studies addressing the loss of axons focused on C-fiber depletion in the epidermis, but little information was obtained regarding myelinated fibers, in which an ultrastructural damage was shown in both experimental animals and patients [Weis et al, 1995; Mizisin et al, 1998]. Electrophysiological studies in diabetic rats have suggested that increased sensory input from myelinated afferents plays an important role in diabetic neuropathic pain, and that NGF can have a pivotal function in inducing the increased input [Khan et al, 2002].

Inconsistent results, however, have been obtained for NGF in animal diabetic neuropathy models, depending on animal strains. In particular, the finding of mechanical hypoalgesia, which has been demonstrated in streptozotocin (STZ)-induced diabetic mice, and can be restored by NGF, is in line with the insensate neuropathy occurring in the majority of humans with diabetic neuropathy [Christianson et al, 2007, 2003]. This is in contrast with the tactile allodynia and increased sensitivity shown in STZ-induced diabetic rats. Depletion of capsaicin-sensitive C-fibers in this model does not alter the development of tactile allodynia, supporting the view that A-fibers, as a potential source of NGF, play a relevant role in increased mechanical sensitivity in the latter model like that presenting in some diabetic patients as a potential source of NGF [Khan et al, 2002]. These latter findings stress the complex role played by NGF in diabetic neuropathy.

In contrast with the discrepant results obtained in diabetic neuropathy, a local increase of NGF can be hypothesized to underlie several conditions of neuropathic pain, such as post-herpetic neuralgia, cisplatinum and taxol-induced neuropathies, as well as post-traumatic injury to peripheral nerves, DRG or spinal cord [Anand, 2004]. If NGF levels are acutely reduced in injured nerve trunks, in these neuropathic painful conditions, skin hyperalgesia and allodynia may be due to a marked local increase of this NT.

The majority of preclinical models that have been developed for neuropathic pain are traumatic injury models (sciatic constriction, spinal nerve ligation, sciatic axotomy, ventral root section), and in all of them, an increase of NGF has been detected [Kanaan et al, 1998; Safieh-Garabedian et al, 2002; Talhouk et al, 2004; Woolf et al, 1997; Djouhri et al, 2001; Cruise et al, 2004; Ueda et al, 2002; Krenz &Weaver, 2000; Obata et al, 2004a; Toma et al, 2000; Saban et al, 2002].

Figure 1 displays the main pathophysiological events underlying neuropathic pain involving NGF.

As in inflammatory pain, recent findings indicate that both SP and CGRP are upregulated in a small population of large- and medium-sized primary sensory neurons after peripheral injury (due to the increase of NGF) in some animal models of neuropathic pain [Ruiz & Baños, 2005]. An increase of CGRP and activin A, which act in concert with NGF, has also been shown in nociceptive neurons that are involved in the sensitization of $TRPV_1$ in primary sensory neurons after injury [Xu & Hall, 2007].

Differential expression of TRP receptors has also been confirmed *in vitro* by the addition of NGF to DRG culture [Anand et al, 2004]. This NGF-dependent mechanism can be hypothesized to occur *in vivo* in neuropathic pain. In injured human DRG sensory neurons, co-expression $TRPV_1$ and $TRPV_3$ has also been demonstrated. In models of post-traumatic neuropathy, the accumulation of $TRPV_1$ and $TRPV_3$ in peripheral nerves after injury indicates that these receptors continue to be exported from the ganglion and/or accumulate in the nerve proximal to injury, despite overall reduced support from peripheral trophic factors, e.g., NGF/GDNF. An increased availability of trophic factors to spared nerve fibers may be similar to the finding in the animal model of partial nerve injury, where undamaged fibers have more available NT because of the reduced uptake by damaged fibers. $TRPV_1$-immunoreactive nerves are also present in injured dorsal spinal roots and DH neurons in the spinal cord, but not in ventral roots, while $TRPV_3$ and $TRPV_4$ were detected in spinal cord motor neurons [Facer et al, 2007]. Furthermore, NGF derived from damaged Schwann cells, or infiltrating macrophages at the site of injury enhances the expression of $TRPV_1$ through the p38 MAPK pathway, which can be antagonized by anti-NGF, p38 MAPK inhibitor, or $TRPA_1$ antisense oligodeoxynucleotides [Obata et al, 2005]. In addition, *de novo* expression of P2X3 receptors is induced by NGF in both spinal cord lamina I and outer lamina II and to the ventro-medial afferent bundle beneath the central canal [Ramer et al, 2001]. In contrast with TRP and purinergic receptors, increased voltage-gated sodium channel activity seems to only partially contribute to NGF-induced hyperexcitability in neuropathic pain, according to Okuse et al (1997). The above phenotypic changes of nociceptive sensory neurons due to increased NGF expression are responsible for an increased excitability of nociceptive terminals.

Another mechanism mediated by increased levels of NGF is the collateral sprouting of sensory neurons, specifically the A-δ-axons involved in nociception and the C-fiber mediating heat nociception, which is antagonized by anti-NGF antibodies, and is responsible for the expansion of pinch and heat field in the skin innervated by damaged neurons [Diamond et al, 1992].

Sympathetic sprouting within axotomized DRGs may also contribute to neuropathic pain. This is related to upregulation of NGF, which is retrogradely transported in the DRG in uninjured sensory axons, and its overexpression, at least in the CCI model, is driven by a glial protein promoter (GFAP) [Ramer et al, 1997, 1998].

In models of thermal injury-induced mechanical hyperalgesia, which mimics the prolonged duration of clinical burn injury pain, NGF was elevated in burn-injured tissue and produced mechanical hyperalgesia [Summer et al, 2006]. It also activated PKC-epsilon, a key mediator in inflammatory and neuropathic pain. This was confirmed by the evidence that intrathecal administration of antisense oligodeoxynucleotides to TrkA and PKC-epsilon, starting 3 days before inducing a burn injury, caused a dose-related decrease of burn-induced primary mechanical hyperalgesia. In addition, intradermal injection of a PKC-epsilon-selective inhibitor eliminated hyperalgesia, supporting the potential usefulness of strategies directed against receptors or downstream pathways activated by NGF as analgesics in pain due to burn injury in humans.

NGF, like NT-3, GDNF and BDNF, has also been implicated in marked and long-lasting mechanical hypernociception following brachial plexus avulsion (BPA). Antibodies against all the above NTs, including NGF, were, in fact, able to post-pone its development in mice when administered locally, systemically or intrathecally at the time of surgery [Quintão et al, 2008].

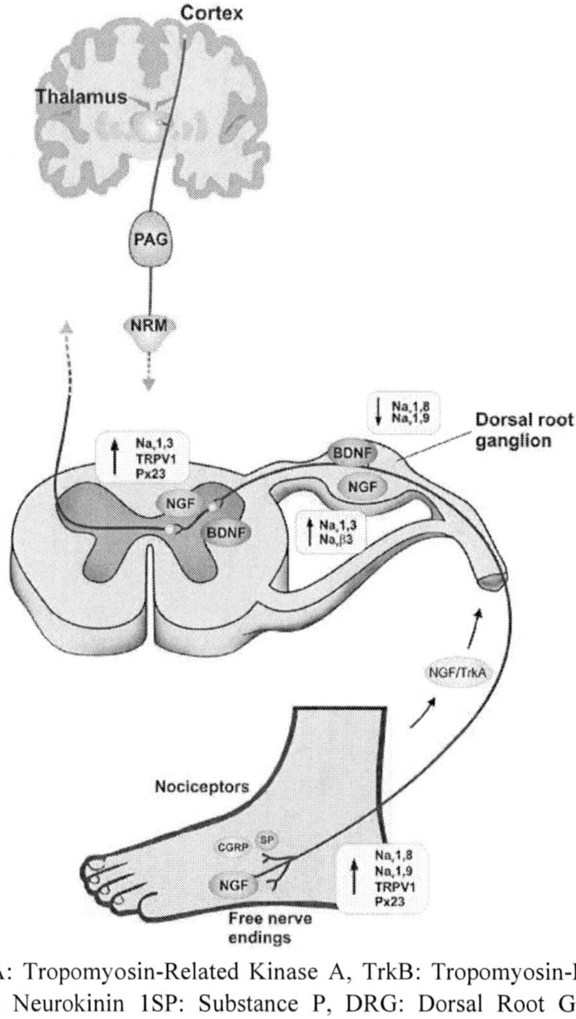

Legend: TrkA: Tropomyosin-Related Kinase A, TrkB: Tropomyosin-Related Kinase B, NK1: Neurokinin 1SP: Substance P, DRG: Dorsal Root Ganglion, PAG: periaqueductal gray region; NRM: magnus raphae nucleus, CGRP: Calcitonin Gene Related Peptide, DH: Dorsal Horn, MAPK:Mitogen-Activated Protein Kinase, ERK: Extracellular Signal-Regulated kinases, CREB: cAMP responsive element binding protein, NR1: subunit 1 of N-methyl-D-aspartic acid receptor, NR2: subunit 2 of N-methyl-D-aspartic acid receptor, NMDA: N-methyl-D-aspartic acid, BDNF Brain-Derived Neurotrophic Factor, NGF: Nerve Growth Factor, TRPV1: Transient receptor potential vanilloid 1.

Figure 1. Potential mechanisms of NGF in the pathophysiological events underlying neuropatic pain. The figure illustrates the modifications induced by NGF released by inflammatory cells, Schawann cells and keratinocytes surrounding the injured nociceptive terminals in the case of neuropathic pain. NGF interacts with own high affinity receptors TRkA on nociceptive neurons . By this interaction it stimulates the release and the synthesis of the sensory neuropeptides SP and CGRP. These peptides are released both in periphery and in spinal cord DH neurons where they interact with their own receptors, NK1 and CGRP receptors, on second order nociceptive neurons. The most significant changes which occur in peripheral nociceptive neurons as a consequence of NGF are: an upregulation of Na^+ channel subunits Nav 1.3 (tipo III), a redistribution of Na^+ channel subunits Nav 1.8 e Nav 1.9 from the somata to the axons of nocieptive neurons and an increase in the auxillary subunit of Na^+ β3 channel. An enhanced responsiveness of TRPV1 is also induced by increasing its phosphorylation. An increased excitability of nociceptive neurons follows the above modifications within the DRG and nerve root; where NGF induces BDNF synthesis through interaction TrkA and intracellular ERK-MAPK pathway activation. The BDNF is transported and released in the DH where interacts with its specific receptor TRkB on second-order neurons. This neurotrophin has a variety of postsynaptic effects. It induces a rapid increase in TrkA phosphorylation and an increase of *c-fos*, *c-jun*, and *krox 24* expression, and of cAMP responsive element binding protein (CREB) phosphorylation, as well as phosphorylation of the mitogen-activated kinase ERK in second-order nociceptors which are important steps in the development of central sensitization underlying pain maintenance. A further effect contributing to central sensitization due to the TrkB phosphorylation, is the increase of NMDA-mediated responses. This increase is due to the phosphorylation of NR1 and NR2B subunits which enhance a three-fold increase in NMDA receptor open time.

As a consequence of increased expression of NGF, TrkA expression was elevated and *c-fos* was upregulated in the spinal DH. If *c-fos* expression plays a crucial role in the development of hyperalgesia in the early stages of neuropathic pain, TrkA receptors may, instead, be involved in the long-lasting adaptive changes of the central pathway in neuropathic pain, as suggested by findings in the CCI sciatic nerve model in rats [Wan et al, 2005].

In addition, in models of both inflammatory pain induced by CFA and neuropathic pain due to axotomy, the enhancement in mechanical allodynia related to the increase of NGF has been shown to be associated with the increase in ERK phosphorylation in TrkA-expressing small- and medium-size neurons. This increase was inhibited by MAPK 1/2 inhibitor, U0126, and was mediated through Trk receptors, because intrathecal treatment with the Trk inhibitor, K252a, reduced the activation of ERK, whose labelling occurred through P2X3 receptors in the terminals [Noguchi et al, 2004]. Likewise, activation of the MAPK pathway in primary nociceptive afferents may be involved in the pathophysiological mechanisms of inflammation-induced radiculopathy or transaction-induced neuropathy, which can be potential targets for pharmacological intervention [Obata et al, 2004b].

It has been demonstrated that, after an inflammatory insult as well as sciatic nerve transection, NGF synthesized within the nerve root and DRG induces BDNF expression through TrkA receptors and intracellular ERK-MAPK pathway activation [Obata et al, 2004b].

The crucial role played by BDNF in neuropathic pain is, furthermore, supported by the demonstration that the local inactivation of this NT decreases the incidence and the severity of autotomy and neuroma formation, but did not influence neuron regeneration [Marcol et al, 2007].

BDNF also contributes to the increased excitability of spinal dorsal neurons, as shown in models of CCI and underlies central sensitization related to neuropathic pain [Lu et al, 2007]. Actions of BDNF on excitatory synaptic drive to putative excitatory, 'delay' firing neurons in the substantia gelatinosa, which are exclusively presynaptic and involve increased miniature excitatory postsynaptic current (mEPSC) frequency and amplitude without changes in the function of postsynaptic AMPA receptors. In contrast, BDNF exerts both pre- and postsynaptic actions on 'tonic' cells. These selective and differential actions of BDNF on excitatory and inhibitory neurons contributes to the global increase in DH network excitability, as assessed by the amplitude of depolarization-induced increases in intracellular Ca^{2+} [Lu et al, 2007].

In recent years, emerging evidence has suggested that NGF, other than regulating sensory neuron phenotype by elevating expression of ion channels and receptors, is able to upregulate the number and efficacy of sensory μ opioid receptors (MORs), which are colocalized with CGRP, TrkA and p75 receptors within DRG, rendering sites of painful inflammation more susceptible to better pain control. These findings support the potential of this NT to overcome the unresponsiveness to opioids of certain neuropathic pain states [Mousa et al, 2007].

Chapter 5

PATHOPHYSIOLOGICAL MECHANISMS OF MIGRAINE

Neurobiological, genetic and advanced brain imaging studies have provided new insights into migraine pathogenesis. Basic concepts of migraine pathophysiology include: (i) an altered neuronal excitability during the interictal phase; (ii) biochemical abnormalities outside attacks involving serotonergic, dopaminergic, and noradrenergic systems; (iii) cortical spreading depression as the basis of aura; (iv) trigeminovascular activation that accounts for the headache phase; and (v) activation of the periacqueductal gray matter (PAG) as a putative "migraine generator or modulator", which may explain some aspects of central sensitization or change in phenotypic expression of the disorder from an episodic to a chronic form [Sanchez-Del-Rio et al, 2006; Cutrer & Huerter, 2007; Silberstein, 2004; Dodick & Silberstein, 2006; Diener & May, 1996; May & Matharu, 2007].

In the last few years a great body of experimental evidence has supported the occurrence of a peripheral sensitization of trigeminal nociceptive afferents innervating the intracranial blood vessels and meninges as the first event that accounts for the pulsating/throbbing head pain during a migraine attack and the associated increase in intracranial sensitivity [Malick & Burstein, 2000]. This results in the aggravation of pain by mechanical stimuli such as those produced by the small increases in intracranial pressure due to coughing or bending.

Peripheral sensitization of trigeminal nociceptive neurons may be induced by the release of algogenic or inflammatory substances from various sources, including these same neurons after their activation. Some of these substances, such as IL-1β, IL-6, TNF-α and PAF can contribute to NGF release from peripheral trigeminal endings [Burstein, 2001]. This inflammatory component associated with trigeminovascular activation is supported by the demonstration of an upregulation of proinflammatory cytokines, such as IL-1β, IL-6 and TNF-α, which have been recognized to play a pivotal role in the experimental model of neurogenic inflammation [DeLeo & Yezierski, 2001].

Experimental data also suggest that NGF activates mast cells through the collaborative interaction with lysophosphatidyl serine expressed on the membrane of activated platelets. This could be of relevance for neurogenic inflammation subsequent to trigeminovascular system activation [Levy et al, 2006; Sugiyama et al, 1985; Kawamoto et al, 2002; Bonini et al, 2003].

Furthermore, the development of a delayed inflammatory response in the context of neurogenic inflammation consequent to trigeminal activation has been emphasized in a rat model of meningeal inflammation due to a brief nitroglycerin infusion, by the findings of a dose-dependent Type II inducible NO synthase (iNOS) mRNA up-regulation in dura mater macrophages and the increase in the corresponding protein expression at 4, 6 and 10 hours after infusion. Consistent with development of a delayed inflammatory response, IL-1β in dura mater and IL-6 in dural macrophages and CSF were detected [Reuter et al, 2001]. In a more recent study, carried out in the same model, the increase in iNOS expression was preceded by a significant increase in nuclear factor-kappaB (NF-κB) activity, due to the reduction in the inhibitory protein-κ-Bα (IκBα) and the upregulation of NF-κB [Reuter et al, 2002]. In agreement with these experimental data, the transitory increase in levels of the proinflammatory cytokines IL-1β, IL-6 and TNF-α was demonstrated by our group in the internal jugular blood of migraine without aura patients assessed in the early phase of the attack. These elevated levels were associated with an increase in intracellular adhesion molecule 1 (ICAM-1) and a significant increase in NF-κB activity preceding the increase in iNOS expression in mononuclear cells [Sarchielli et al, 2006a, 2006b]. A transient increase in PAF levels was also detected in the internal jugular blood of migraine patients during attacks [Sarchielli et al, 2004b].

All the above substances are part of the "inflammatory soup" that can activate meningeal trigeminal nociceptive neurons. In this context, NGF induced by proinflammatory cytokines and PAF can directly sensitize nociceptive neurons through rapid modulation of heat/vanilloid receptors or by up-regulating ion channels, with particular regard to those involved in TTX-s and TTX-r Na^+ currents [Cummins et al, 2007; Padilla et al, 2007; Fabbretti et al, 2006].

The repetitive activation of trigeminal endings induces an activity- or use-dependent neuronal plasticity of trigeminal nociceptive neurons. This modifies their subsequent performance, enabling normally innocuous inputs to activate them (allodynia) and determining exaggerated or prolonged responses to noxious inputs (hyperalgesia) [Sarchielli et al, 2007a]. This central neuronal activation results in temporal summation of nociceptive responses. More specifically, the activity-dependent plasticity is the consequence of the summation of C-fiber-evoked slow synaptic currents produced by glutamate acting on NMDA and metabotropic glutamate receptors (mGluRs), and neuropeptides, such as CGRP and SP, as well as by the recruitment of postsynaptic voltage-gated Ca^{2+} plateau currents and release of BDNF. Increased synaptic and voltage-gated currents contribute to a use-dependent facilitation (*wind-up*) of trigeminal nociceptors during repetitive C-fiber inputs by producing nonlinear cumulative depolarizations lasting tens of seconds [Vikelis & Mitsikostas, 2007; Dodick & Silberstein, 2006]. These events are responsible for a progressive increase in the amount of pain experienced and underlie the early stages of central sensitization, which are interfaced with a later stage in which a cascade of intracellular biochemical events leads to longer lasting changes in the properties of trigeminal nociceptive neurons.

Chapter 6

PATHOPHYSIOLOGY OF FIBROMYALGIA

Fibromyalgia syndrome (FM) is a chronic pain syndrome defined as a widespread pain for more than 3 months and the presence of >11 of 18 tender points [Wolfe et al, 1990]. It represents the extreme of a wide spectrum of musculo-skeletal pain syndromes, which mostly affects women with a ratio of 9:1 to men [Wolfe et al, 1990]. The majority of studies concerning FM patients have shown abnormalities of pain sensitivity using different methods of sensory testing. A generalized lowering of pressure pain thresholds in FM patients and a mechanical pain hypersensitivity (allodynia) of FM patients not limited to tender points but diffusely widespread are common features [Petzke et al, 2003].

Pain in FM is consistently felt in the musculature and has been related to the sensitization of both peripheral and CNS pain pathways [Price & Staud, 2005; Staud & Rodriguez, 2006].

Accumulating evidence suggests that peripheral impulse input from deep tissues and joints plays an important role in FM patients. The most significant findings point to relevant alterations in skin and muscles. They include the presence of ragged red fibers and moth-eaten fibers, inflammatory infiltrates and DNA fragmentation in affected muscles, muscle perfusion deficits confirmed by the reduction in pH (related to ischemia), reduction in phosphorylation potential, and in total oxidative capacity [Averill et al, 1986; Jacobsen et al, 1991; Kalyan-Raman et al, 1984; Bengtsson et al, 1986]. An increase in inflammatory mediators and proinflammatory cytokines as well as advanced glycation end products has also been demonstrated [Hoheisel et al, 1998; Wallace et al, 2001; Giovengo et al, 1999]. All these biochemical mediators induce changes in the properties of muscle primary nociceptive afferents underlying their peripheral sensitization. The consequent maintained tonic impulse input from muscles contributes to the development of central sensitization [Arendt-Nielsen et al, 2003; Sorensen et al, 1998]. In this condition, the long-term neuroplastic changes in DH neurons exceed the antinociceptive capabilities of affected patients, resulting in ever-increasing pain sensitivity and spontaneous pain. Nociceptive activity in the peripheral tissues of FM patients, however, does not necessarily have to be extensive, because central sensitization requires little sustained input to maintain the sensitized state and chronic pain.

From a clinical point of view, allodynia for cutaneous/muscle mechanical stimulation and hyperalgesia for electrical as well as thermal stimulation, support the occurrence of central sensitization in FM patients [Price et al, 2002; Staud et al, 2003]. They have also been shown to display enhanced temporal summation of heat-evoked second pain compared to pain-free controls [Price et al, 2002; Staud et al, 2003]. Recent research clearly confirmed in these patients enhanced pain sensitivity, with lower stimulus intensities needed to establish *wind-up* and lower stimulus frequencies to maintain it than in controls [Staud et al, 2001, 2004]. In addition, *wind-up* after-sensations are greatly prolonged, indirectly suggesting that *wind-up* is abnormally maintained in FM [Staud et al, 2001, 2004]. Abnormal *wind-up*, prolonged after-sensations, and mechanical allodynia are, therefore, the result of abnormal nociceptive input from the periphery and abnormal central pain mechanisms relative to controls. They represent peculiar features of central sensitization that have been found to be relevant predictors of clinical pain in FM [Price & Staud, 2005; Staud & Rodriguez, 2006]. Pain-related negative affects have been shown to significantly contribute to pain in these pathological conditions [Price & Staud, 2005; Staud & Rodriguez, 2006].

Chapter 7

INVOLVEMENT OF NGF IN THE PATHOPHYSIOLOGICAL MECHANISMS OF MIGRAINE AND FIBROMYALGIA

Localization studies outlined the pivotal contribution of NGF signaling to nociception of trigeminal neurons. NGF has been demonstrated in these neurons to be effective in enhancing capsaicin and K^+ evoked CGRP release [Price et al, 2005]. This action, together with activation of the ERK pathway, is mediated by stimulation of the CGRP promoter. NGF has also been demonstrated to increase functional activities of the $TRPA_1$ channel and P2X3 receptors. This leads to plastic changes in the trigeminal nociceptive pathways mediating head pain [Price et al, 2005; Diogenes et al, 2007; Simonetti et al, 2006], which is counteracted by anti-NGF treatment [D'Arco et al, 2007].

These observations outlined the relevance of NGF in trigeminal pain and prompted research aimed at determining its levels in migraine. The more relevant pathophysiological mechanisms of migraine involving NGF are shown in figure 2.

NGF measurements in the peripheral blood of CM patients showed reduced levels that were attributed to altered platelet turnover of this NT [Blandini et al, 2005]. Further research, however, carried out on patients with chronic daily headache (CDH) with a previous history of episodic migraine without aura and, more recently, on patients suffering from CM diagnosed according to the current International Classification Headache Disorders (ICHD-II) criteria [Subcommittee of the International Headache Society, 2004], suggests the implication of NGF in the maintenance of chronic head pain.

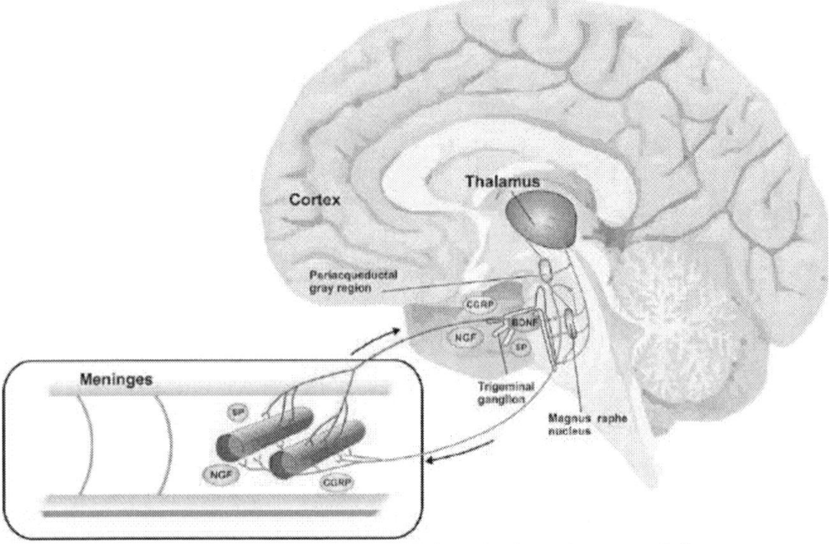

Legend: TG: trigeminal ganglion, TNC: trigeminal nucleus caudalis, NGF: Nerve Growth Factor, TrkA: Tropomyosin-Related Kinase A, CGRP:Calcitonin Gene Related Peptide, NKA: Neurokinin-A, PAF: Platelet Activating Factor, 5HT: 5-hydroxytryptamine, DH: Dorsal Horn, P2X3: Purinergic receptor P2X, ligand-gated ion channel, 3, BDNF: Brain-derived neurotrophic factor, TRPV1: transient potential receptor vanilloid 1, NMDA: N-methyl-D-aspartic acid.

Figure 2. Relevance of NGF in the pathophysiological mechanisms of migraine. Activation of nociceptive afferent fibers of trigeminal ganglion (TG) neurons innervating the meningeal blood vessels and the subsequent activation of second-order dorsal horn neurons in the trigeminal nucleus caudalis (TNC) is the main mechanism underlying migraine headache. In the meninges, NGF released by activated mastcells, is responsible of the release of vasoactive neuropeptides CGRP and NKA, by interacting with own high affinity receptor TrkA on trigeminal terminals. There are also other molecules contributing to the release of these peptides, belonging to the so called inflammatory soup (K+, PAF, bradikinin, 5HT, some proinflammatory cytokines) which contributes to neurogenic vasodilation of meningeal vessels. Sensory neuropeptides are also anterogradely transported and released in the DH by the central terminals of the first-order nociceptors interacting with second-order dorsal horn neurons. NGF also induce the *de novo* synthesis of sensory neuropeptides and up-regulate P2X3 and TRPV1 receptors. It also induce the synthesis of BDNF in the TGN form which this latter neurotrophin is anterogradely transported and released from the central terminals of trigeminal nociceptors in the TNC. Through interaction with own receptor TrkB, BDNF increases the excitability of TNC neurons, also by stimulate glutamatergic transmission via enhancement of NMDA receptor functioning. Through the same post-synaptic mechanisms described for neuropathic pain it intervenes in central sensitization which is involved in head pain maintenance and chronification.

The first of these studies, carried out by our group, investigated NGF levels in the CSF of a group of CDH patients comparing them with those of an age- and sex-matched control group. This latter group included subjects for whom CSF and blood examinations as well as adequate instrumental investigations excluded CNS or systemic diseases. Values of SP and CGRP were also determined and were significantly correlated with NGF levels in the CSF of both CDH patients and controls. Significantly higher CSF levels of NGF, SP and CGRP were detected without significant differences between patients with symptomatic drug overuse and those without. A significant correlation also emerged in the same study between NGF levels and the duration of chronic headache and number of days with headache per month [Sarchielli et al, 2001].

If the evidence of increased CSF levels of NGF confirmed the pivotal role of this NT in CDH patients, the concomitant increase in the levels of sensory neuropeptides of trigeminal origin, SP and CGRP, supported the intervention of NGF in enhancing their synthesis, transport, content and release from trigeminal nociceptive neurons in the same patients, as shown in animal pain models [Sarchielli et al, 2001].

In a subsequent study, levels of NGF and those of another NGF-dependent NT, BDNF, as well as glutamate were determined in the CSF of a further group of patients affected by CDH with a previous history of episodic migraine [Sarchielli et al, 2002]. Significantly higher levels of both NGF and BDNF were found in CDH patients compared with controls. Glutamate levels were also significantly higher than those of controls. Levels of the two NTs were significantly correlated with each other and with levels of glutamate in the patient group. As in the previous study, no significant differences were found in BDNF, NGF and glutamate levels between CDH patients with analgesic abuse and those without.

These findings concur with those obtained in experimental pain models, which demonstrated that the nociceptive effect of NGF seems to be exerted through the upregulation of BDNF mRNA and protein in TrkA nociceptive neurons. In contrast, BDNF release is responsible for increased synaptic activity through the potentiation of glutamatergic transmission, as suggested by the increase in glutamate levels in the CSF of our CDH patients. The increase in glutamatergic transmission is believed to underlie central sensitization, thus playing a pivotal role in the maintenance of head pain in these patients.

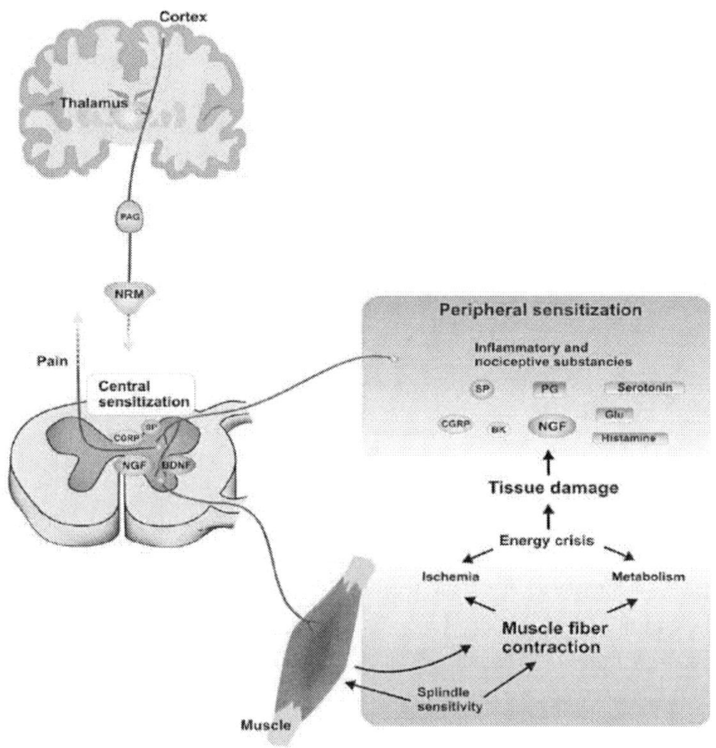

Legend: NGF: nerve growth factor; SP: Substance P; CGRP: calcitonin-gene related peptide; TrkA: Tropomyosin-Related Kinase A, TrkB: Tropomyosin-Related Kinase B, BK: bradykinin; PAG: periaqueductal gray region; NRM: magnus raphae nucleus, BDNF Brain-Derived Neurotrophic Factor. NMDA: N-methyl-D-asparate receptor; DH: Dorsal Horn, ERK: Extracellular Signal-Regulated kinases, MAPK: Mitogen-Activated Protein Kinase.

Figure 3. Potential mechanisms of NGF in the pathophysiological events underlying fibromyalgia. Abnormalities in skin and muscles have been demonstrated in fibromyalgia which include an increase of proinflammatory cytokines and excitatory amino acids, a release of SP in muscle tissue, DNA fragmentation within muscle cells, and muscle perfusion deficits. In this condition NGF can be released by inflammatory cells, Schwann cells and keratinocytes and interacts with own high affinity receptors TRkA on nociceptive neurons. By this way it stimulates the release and synthesis of the sensory neuropeptides SP and CGRP both in periphery and in DH, increasing excitability of first and second-order neurons. Like in the case of neuropathic pain, NGF also induces in DRG, BDNF expression through TrkA and intracellular ERK-MAPK pathway activation. BDNF is transported and released in the DH where interacts with its on receptor TRkB on second-order neurons contributing to central sensitization by enhancing glutamatergic transmission, underlying widespread pain sensation in fibromyalgia.

Based on the above results, we hypothesized that similar mechanisms could be implicated in other chronic painful conditions, such as FM. The most relevant pathophysiological mechanisms involving NGF are displayed in Figure 3. Based on this assumption, we therefore assessed NGF and BDNF levels in the CSF of patients with primary FM syndrome and compared results obtained in the CSF with those of patients with CM, diagnosed according to the current ICHD-II criteria, and those of control subjects [Sarchielli et al, 2007b]. The relationship between these levels and the duration of chronic pain and quantitative pain measures in both patient groups was also assessed. As in our previous research, we found significantly higher levels of NGF, BDNF and glutamate in patients with CM. The same levels were also increased in patients with primary FM syndrome. The findings of an increase in NGF levels in the CSF concurs, in particular, with results of a previous study from Giovengo et al [1999], demonstrating increased concentration of this NT compared to controls although with a greater variability.

Although accumulating evidence suggests that pain is maintained by tonic impulse input from deep tissues, such as muscle and joints in combination with central sensitization mechanisms in FM [Saragovi et al, 2000], no correlation was found between quantitative sensory testing measures and glutamate as well as BDNF and NGF levels in the CSF of our FM patients. This was also true for patients with CM.

The involvement of NGF in both chronic pathological conditions leads to the hypothesis that its increase is not a specific feature of CM, since it could be detected in other chronic painful conditions intervening in common mechanisms underlying the pathogenic basis of pain perpetuation. Furthermore, the rise in NGF levels seems to be related to pain *per se* because it is not influenced by analgesic or anti-inflammatory drug abuse.

Chapter 8

Potential of NGF Targeting Strategies in Neuropathic Pain, Chronic Migraine and Fibromyalgia

A growing body of evidence suggests the anti-hyperalgesic effect of pharmacological interference with NGF-TrkA interactions in inflammatory and neuropathic pain [Saragovi et al, 2000; Hefti et al, 2006; Gwak et al, 2003; Salter, 2005; Koltzenburg et al, 1999; Wild et al, 2007; Ro et al, 1999; Christiansen & Hulschboch, 1997; Halvorson et al, 2005; Chudler et al, 1997; Jimenez-Andrade et al, 2007].

NGF-neutralizing antibodies were also able to attenuate mechanical and thermal hyperalgesia following spinal cord injury or CCI sciatic nerve [Ro et al, 1999], which corresponds, at a molecular level, to a decrease in CGRP density in the spinal cord (laminae I to IV) [Christiansen & Hulschboch, 1997]. In addition, the subcutaneous infusion of a synthetic TrkA–IgG fusion protein, which binds NGF with high-affinity capacity, produced a slow reduction in CGRP and $TRPV_1$ expression by sensory neurons [Xue et al, 2007]. Furthermore, autoimmunization of rodents with NGF reduced Nav 1.8 mRNA expression and TTX-r Na^+ currents in appropriate sensory neurons [Chudler et al, 1997].

NGF-neutralizing antibodies have been demonstrated to exert an analgesic effect greater than that achieved with acute administration of 10 or 30 mg/kg morphine in an experimental model of bone-cancer pain [Halvorson et al, 2005]. This therapy also reduced some neurochemical changes associated with peripheral and central sensitization in DRG and spinal cord, without influencing disease progression or markers of sensory and sympathetic innervation in the skin or bone [Sevcik et al, 2005].

More recently, monoclonal antibodies against NGF have been used as novel NGF sequestering therapies [Cattaneo et al, 1999]. They were tested in a skeletal pain model in mouse due to fracture where pain was reversed by 10mg/kg morphine [Jimenez-Andrade et al, 2007]. In this model, monoclonal anti-NGF antibodies reduced fracture-induced pain-related behaviors by over 50%. Treatment with anti-NGF antibodies also decreased *c-fos* and dynorphin upregulation in the spinal cord at day 2 post-fracture but not p-ERK and *c-fos* expression at 20 and 90 min, respectively, suggesting the involvement of this NT in the maintenance but not in the acute generation of such type of pain. While anti-NGF antibodies do not significantly cross the blood-brain barrier, it can be hypothesized that their anti-hyperalgesic effect is due to the blockade of the activation and/or sensitization of the CGRP/TrkA positive fibers that normally represent the majority of sensory fibers innervating bone.

Anti-NGF antibodies have been recently demonstrated to reduce some, but not all, signs of the complex regional pain syndrome (CRPS) I-like in a rat fracture model. They reduced neuropeptide levels in sciatic nerve and nociceptive sensitization in the anti-NGF treated animals. Conversely, anti-NGF antibodies did not decrease hindpaw edema, warmth or cytokine production, suggesting the complexity of the mechanism of CRPS pathogenesis in which only some aspects seem to be related to NGF up-regulation and signaling [Sabsovich et al, 2007].

Functional neutralization of the TrkA receptor using NGF-sequestering molecules is another approach to antagonize NGF action targeting the signaling transduction pathways depending on receptor activation. One such molecule, MNAC13, a monoclonal antibody, has been demonstrated to display a high affinity and specificity for the NGF receptor TrkA, and a neutralizing activity toward the NGF/TrkA interaction [Cattaneo et al, 1999; Covaceuszach, 2001, 2005]. Treatment with the MNAC13 anti-TrkA antibody impairs TrkA signaling, resulting in the inhibition of SHC-mediated as well as phospholipase Cy (PLCγ) pathways [Ugolini et al, 2007]. This monoclonal antibody has been tested in the formalin-evoked pain licking responses in mice, where it produced a significant antiallodynic effect. The same antiallodynic effect and a remarkable functional recovery were observed in mice subjected to sciatic nerve ligation, with effects persisting after administration [Ugolini et al, 2007].

Non peptidergic molecules with antagonistic properties, such as compound PD90780 [Colquhoun et al, 2004; Spiegel et al, 1995] and kynurenic acid derivatives [Jarvis et al, 1997] have been shown to prevent the binding of NGF on low-affinity p75 receptors, but their use has not been assessed in animal pain models.

More recently, a novel nonpeptidic molecule, ALE-0540, has been demonstrated not to prevent the binding of NGF to the p75 receptor but to specifically inhibit the binding of NGF to TrkA. By preventing TrkA phosphorylation, ALE-0540 not only antagonizes the signal transduction pathway and biological responses mediated by this receptor but also blocks both neuropathic and thermally-induced inflammatory pain. Furthermore, in the L5/L6 ligation model of neuropathic pain in rats, both systemic and intrathecal administration of ALE-0540 produced an antiallodynic effect [Owolabi et al, 1999]. This promising nonpeptidic small molecule opens, therefore, new perspectives in the development of agents for the treatment of pain. The pharmacological and safety profile of this first non peptidergic NGF receptor antagonist molecule revealed the lack of interaction with known analgesic targets, including histamine 1, endothelin A, 5-HT_2, cannabinoids and opioid (μ, δ, and k) receptors reflecting the lack of central side effects of these compounds.

Further NGF mimetics with antagonistic action were produced with potential clinical applications. In particular, small monomeric cyclic analogs miming the β-turn regions of NGF were designed and synthesized [LeSauteur et al, 1995]. Among them, potent competitive antagonists were derived from the NGF β-turn C-D, which inhibits NGF binding to TrkA receptors and neurite outgrowth in PC12 cells. Until now, these analogues were used to study the biological and receptor binding properties of NGF but they have never been tested in animal pain models. A small peptide named C (92-96) that blocks NGF-TrkA interactions, in particular, was studied for it effects on cortex cholinergic synapses and has been demonstrated to induce a significant decrease in the size of vesicular acetylcholine transporter-immunoreactive sites [Debeir et al, 1999]. The use of this approach for modulating and reducing molecular and neuronal events underlying chronic pain can be hypothesized from a theoretical point of view. However, it opens the question of the dependency on NGF of correct functioning of the CNS and the potential impact of this treatment on the correct maintenance of synaptic contacts and functioning in the adult CNS, which may not be limited to cholinergic neurons [Hulsebosch et al, 1988; Garofalo et al, 1992].

Studies in animal pain models in which TrkA immunoadhesins are administered have shown that sequestering of endogenous NGF is able to block the hyperalgesia associated with inflammation [Katsura et al, 2006].

However, these large molecules are unlikely to be clinically useful. Therefore, efforts have been recently directed to identify small molecule agonists/antagonists based on crystal structure of the NGF-TrkAd5 complex, taking into account the biochemical evidence supporting the involvement of domain 5 of the TrkA receptor in the binding of NGF. TrkAd5 has been shown to be efficacious in preclinical models of inflammatory pain by the sequestration of excess levels of endogenous NGF, and therefore, represents a novel therapeutic agent for chronic pain conditions in which an inflammatory component can be recognized [Dawbarn et al, 2006].

In the last few years, there has also been a growing interest in new targets for pain therapy among NGF intracellular signaling pathways. Activation of PKC could be one of these potential targets even in NGF hyperalgesia [Khasar et al, 1999]. A PKC ε selective inhibitor peptide or related compounds have been proposed for the treatment of chronic pain states, but need to be tested in animals before use in human painful conditions.

Despite the promising strategies against NGF, it is currently difficult to define the potential role of anti-NGF strategies in neuropathic conditions. As already shown in some experimental models, NGF was helpful in favoring the regeneration of damaged sensory neurons. This furnished the rationale for the use of this NF in the treatment of diabetic or HIV-induced neuropathies, which failed, however, to demonstrate any significant clinical efficacy.

Neotrofin, an interesting molecule that enhances endogenous NGF levels, has been recently developed to prevent phenotypic, functional and structural changes occurring in diabetic neuropathy, by antagonizing the depletion of NGF protein. This effect was accompanied by the maintenance of normal nerve levels of the sensory neuropeptides SP and CGRP. Thermal hypoalgesia and conduction slowing of large sensory fibers in diabetic rats were ameliorated by neotrofin treatment, which had no effect on conduction slowing in large motor fibers or on reduced myelinated fiber axonal caliber. Therefore, the use of small molecules able to enhance endogenous production of NGF may be a promising alternative to either exogenous treatment with neurotrophic factors or gene therapy as a therapeutic approach to treat some neuropathies characterized by sensory loss, in particular diabetic neuropathy. Future trials on these small molecules are warranted [Calcutt et al, 2006].

Despite the above observations, the majority of studies on NGF antagonism in animal models of neuropathic pain have focused only on the prevention of hyperalgesia and allodynia after injury. In a recent study, in particular, the effects of anti-NGF antibodies in models of neuropathic and inflammatory pain inflammation, spinal nerve ligation and STZ-induced neuropathic pain models were assessed from approximately day 3 to day 7 after treatment. A significant effect on thermal hyperalgesia was observed only in the spinal nerve ligation model. In the mouse CCI model, monoclonal anti-NGF antibodies were able to decrease tactile allodynia when administered 2 weeks after surgery. Repeated administration of this antibody to CCI in mice for 3 weeks produced a sustained reversal (from day 4 to day 21) of tactile allodynia that was restored 5 days after the end of administration. Based on the above results, NGF antagonists, such as fully human monoclonal anti-NGF antibodies, can be hypothesized to have a potential therapeutic utility, at least in some human neuropathic pain conditions, with no development of tolerance to antagonism [Wild et al, 2007].

The only anti-TrkA monoclonal antibody with functional neutralizing properties, MNAC13, has been clearly shown to induce analgesia not only in inflammatory pain but also in neuropathic pain models (formalin-evoked pain-licking responses and sciatic nerve ligation, respectively), with a surprisingly long-lasting effect in the latter. Furthermore, a clear synergistic effect was observed when MNAC13 was administered in combination with opioids at doses that were not efficacious *per se*. These findings provide, therefore, a direct demonstration that strategies based on neutralizing antibodies directed against the TrkA receptor may display potent analgesic effects that should be tested in future research [Ugolini et al, 2007].

In a recent approach, NGF-mimetic peptides were used that were based on chemical modification of amino acid residues at loop 1, loop 4, and the N-terminal region of the NGF molecule as the most relevant for its biological activity. One of these peptides with the highest *in vitro* activity (L1L4), demonstrated by induction of DRG differentiation and tyrosine phosphorylation of TrkA receptor stimulation, has been shown to reduce neuropathic behavior and restore neuronal function in a rat model of peripheral neuropathic pain, thereby suggesting a putative therapeutic role [Colangelo et al, 2008].

Evidence of the involvement of NGF in the pathophysiology of chronic pain and the effort in the development of molecules targeting this NT open, therefore, new insight into the identification of novel therapeutic strategies for the treatment of chronic painful conditions, including inflammatory and neuropathic pain. Much research, however, is needed for evaluating their real application in humans in these pathological conditions.

Chapter 9

CONCLUSIONS

The potential usefulness of anti-NGF treatment in migraine despite recent findings outlining the relevant contribution of NGF signaling to trigeminal nociceptive neurons still remains to be established. Blockade of NGF can be hypothesized as a novel, analgesic symptomatic approach, whereas the use of anti-NGF strategies as prophylactic treatment is more difficult to postulate due to potential CNS side effects, with the only exception of the chronic form of migraine, refractory to any other prophylactic treatment. In this condition, central sensitization is also sustained by an increase in BDNF induced by NGF and related increase in glutamatergic transmission [Kerr et al, 1999; Bennett, 2001]. Because BDNF may function as a modulator of central sensitization, strategies against this NT can be hypothesized as a novel treatment of persistent pain, including neuropathic pain and resistant migraine. The same is true for FM in which central sensitization is the major pathophysiological mechanism.

In contrast with findings available for NGF targeting treatments, limited data are available concerning BDNF. The sequestration of endogenous BDNF reduced pain-related behavior in two models of inflammatory pain [Kerr et al, 1999] and also in neuropathic pain [Yajima et al, 2002, 2005], which resulted in a depression of spinal ERK activation by 40%. BDNF sequestration, however, did not affect mechanical hyperalgesia induced by peripheral capsaicin administration [Mannion et al, 1999]. In addition, in BDNF knockout mice, this NT has been shown to be required for normal pain sensitivity in the hot plate and formalin tests, which suggests the difficulty involved in identifying antagonizing molecules that are selectively directed against the pathological pain mechanism and with a relevant effect on the treatment of pain [MacQueen et al, 2001].

Therapeutic strategies targeting BDNF (anti-BDNF antibodies or TrkB targeting molecules) should, however, be considered with caution. BDNF, in fact, exerts a dual effect by intervening not only in enhancing glutamate transmission, playing a pivotal role in central sensitization, but also in stimulating GABA release from DH interneurons [Pezet et al, 2002], therefore exerting a potential compensatory mechanism in chronic pain. The two opposite effects of BDNF should be investigated in animal pain models before developing novel strategies targeting this NT, with potential application to inflammatory and neuropathic pain as well as CM and FM.

REFERENCES

Amann, R; Schuligoi, R; Herzeg, G; Donnerer, J. Intraplantar injection of nerve growth factor into the rat hind paw: Local edema and effects on thermal nociceptive threshold. *Pain,* 1996 64, 323–329.

Amaya, F; Shimosato, G; Nagano, M; Ueda, M; Hashimoto, S; Tanaka, Y; Suzuki, H; Tanaka, M. NGF and GDNF differentially regulate TRPV1 expression that contributes to development of inflammatory thermal hyperalgesia. *Eur. J. Neurosci,* 2004 20, 2303-2310.

Amaya, F; Wang, H; Costigan, M; Allchorne, AJ; Hatcher, JP; Egerton, J; Stean, T; Morisset, V; Grose, D; Gunthorpe, MJ; Chessell, IP; Tate, S; Green, PJ; Woolf, CJ. The voltage-gated sodium channel Na(v)1.9 is an effector of peripheral inflammatory pain hypersensitivity. *J. Neurosci,* 2006 26, 12852-12860.

Anand, P. Neurotrophic factors and their receptors in human sensory neuropathies. *Prog. Brain Res,* 2004 146, 477-492.

Anand, U; Otto, WR; Casula, MA; Day, NC; Davis, JB; Bountra, C; Birch, R; Anand, P. The effect of neurotrophic factors on morphology, TRPV1 expression and capsaicin responses of cultured human DRG sensory neurons. *Neurosci. Lett,* 2006 399, 51-56.

Apfel, SC. Nerve growth factor for the treatment of diabetic neuropathy: what went wrong, what went right, and what does the future hold? *Int. Rev. Neurobiol,* 2002 50, 393-413.

Apfel, SC. Neurotrophic factors and diabetic peripheral neuropathy. *Eur. Neurol,* 1999 41, 27-34.

Apfel, SC; Wright, DE; Wiideman, AM; Dormia, C; Snider, WD; Kessler, JA. Nerve growth factor regulates the expression of brain-derived neurotrophic factor mRNA in the peripheral nervous system. *Mol. Cell Neurosci,* 1996 7, 134–142.

Arendt-Nielsen, L; Graven-Nielsen, T. Central sensitization in fibromyalgia and other musculoskeletal disorders. *Curr. Pain Headache Rep,* 2003 7, 355-361.

Arnett, MG; Ryals, JM; Wright, DE. Pro-NGF, sortilin, and p75NTR: potential mediators of injury-induced apoptosis in the mouse dorsal root ganglion. *Brain Res,* 2007 1183, 32-42.

Averill, S; Michael, GJ; Shortland, PJ; Leavesley, RC; King, VR; Bradbury, EJ; McMahon, Bartels EM; Danneskiold-Samsoe, B. Histological abnormalities in muscle from patients with certain types of fibrositis. *Lancet,* 1986 1, 755–757.

Averill, S; Michael, GJ; Shortland, PJ; Leavesley, RC; King, VR; Bradbury, EJ; McMahon, SB; Priestley, JV. NGF and GDNF ameliorate the increase in ATF3 expression which occurs in dorsal root ganglion cells in response to peripheral nerve injury. *Eur. J. Neurosci,* 2004 19, 1437-1445.

Bengtsson, A; Henriksson, KG; Larsson, J. Reduced high-energy phosphate levels in the painful muscles of patients with primary fibromyalgia. *Arthritis Rheum,* 1986 29, 817–821.

Bennett, DL. Neurotrophic factors: important regulators of nociceptive function. *Neuroscientist,* 2001 7, 13-17.

Bienenstock, J; Tomioka, M; Matsuda, H; Stead, RH; Quinonez, G; Simon, GT; Coughlin, MD; Denburg, JA. The role of mast cells in inflammatory processes: evidence for nerve/mast cell interactions. *Int. Arch. Allergy Appl. Immunol,* 1987 82, 238-243.

Blandini, F; Rinaldi, L; Tassorelli, C; Sances, G; Motta, M; Samuele, A; Fancellu, R; Nappi, G; Leon, A. Peripheral levels of BDNF and NGF in primary headaches. *Cephalalgia,* 2006 26, 136-142.

Bonini, S; Rasi, G; Bracci-Laudiero, ML; Procoli, A; Aloe, L. Nerve growth factor: neurotrophin or cytokine? *Int. Arch. Allergy Immunol,* 2003 131, 80-84.

Bowsher, D; Haggett, C. Paradoxical burning sensation produced by cold stimulation in patients with neuropathic pain. *Pain,* 2005 117, 230.

Bracci-Laudiero, L; Aloe, L; Caroleo, MC; Buanne, P; Costa, N; Starace, G; Lundeberg, T. Endogenous NGF regulates CGRP expression in human monocytes, and affects HLA-DR and CD86 expression and IL-10 production. *Blood,* 2005 106, 3507-3514.

Brodie, C. Platelet activating factor induces nerve growth factor production by rat astrocytes. *Neurosci. Lett,* 1995 186, 5-8.

Burstein, R. Deconstructing migraine headache into peripheral and central sensitization. *Pain,* 2001 89, 107-110.

Cahill, CM; Dray, A; Coderre, TJ. Intrathecal nerve growth factor restores opioid effectiveness in an animal model of neuropathic pain. *Neuropharmacology,* 2003 45, 543-552.

Calcutt, NA; Freshwater, JD; Hauptmann, N; Taylor, EM; Mizisin, AP. Protection of sensory function in diabetic rats by Neotrofin. *Eur. J. Pharmacol,* 2006 534, 187-193.

Cattaneo, A; Capsoni, S; Margotti, E; Righi, M;, Kontsekova, E; Pavlik, P; Filipcik, P; Novak, M. Functional blockade of tyrosine kinase A in the rat basal forebrain by a novel antagonistic anti-receptor monoclonal antibody. *J. Neurosci,* 1999 19, 9687-9697.

Chao, MV; Rajagopal, R; Lee, FS. Neurotrophin signalling in health and disease. *Clin Sci (Lond),* 2006 110, 167-173.

Chen, Y; Li, GW; Wang, C; Gu, Y; Huang, LY. Mechanisms underlying enhanced P2X receptor-mediated responses in the neuropathic pain state. *Pain,* 2005 119, 38-48.

Chien, CC; Fu, WM; Huang, HI; Lai, YH; Tsai, YF; Guo, SL; Wu, TJ; Ling, QD. Expression of neurotrophic factors in neonatal rats after peripheral inflammation. *J. Pain,* 2007 8, 161-167.

Christensen, MD; Hulsebosch, CE. Spinal cord injury and anti-NGF treatment results in changes in CGRP density and distribution in the dorsal horn in the rat. *Exp. Neurol,* 1997 147, 463-475.

Christianson, JA; Ryals, JM; Johnson, MS; Dobrowsky, RT; Wright, DE. Neurotrophic modulation of myelinated cutaneous innervation and mechanical sensory loss in diabetic mice. *Neuroscience,* 2007 145, 303-313.

Christianson, JA; Ryals, JM; McCarson, KE; Wright, DE. Beneficial actions of neurotrophin treatment on diabetes-induced hypoalgesia in mice. *J. Pain,* 2003 4, 493-504.

Chudler, EH; Anderson, LC; Byers, MR. Nerve growth factor depletion by autoimmunization produces thermal hypoalgesia in adult rats. *Brain Res,* 1997 765, 327-330.

Colangelo, AM; Bianco, MR; Vitagliano, L; Cavaliere, C; Cirillo, G; De Gioia, L; Diana, D; Colombo, D; Redaelli, C; Zaccaro, L; Morelli, G; Papa, M; Sarmientos, P; Alberghina, L; Martegani, E. A new nerve growth factor-mimetic peptide active on neuropathic pain in rats. *J. Neurosci,* 2008 28, 2698-2709.

Colquhoun, A; Lawrance, GM; Shamovsky, IL; Riopelle, RJ; Ross, GM. Differential activity of the nerve growth factor (NGF) antagonist PD90780 [7-(benzolylamino)-4,9-dihydro-4-methyl-9-oxo-pyrazolo[5,1-b]quinazoline-2-carboxylic acid] suggests altered NGF-p75NTR interactions in the presence of TrkA. *J. Pharmacol. Exp. Ther,* 2004 310, 505-511.

Cortright, DN; Szallasi, A. Biochemical pharmacology of the vanilloid receptor TRPV1. An update. *Eur. J. Biochem*, 2004 271, 1814-1819.

Coutaux, A; Adam, F; Willer, JC; Le Bars, D. Hyperalgesia and allodynia: peripheral mechanisms. *Joint Bone Spine,* 2005 72, 359-371.

Covaceuszach, S; Cattaneo, A; Lamba, D. Neutralization of NGF-TrkA receptor interaction by the novel antagonistic anti-TrkA monoclonal antibody MNAC13: a structural insight. *Proteins,* 2005 58, 717-727.

Covaceuszach, S; Cattaneo, A; Lamba, D. Purification, crystallization and preliminary X-ray analysis of the Fab fragment from MNAC13, a novel antagonistic anti-tyrosine kinase A receptor monoclonal antibody. *Acta Crystall D. Biol. Cruystallog,* 2001 57, 1307-1309.

Créange, A; Barlovatz-Meimon, G; Gherardi, RK. Cytokines and peripheral nerve disorders. *Eur. Cytokine Netw,* 1997 8, 145-151.

Cruise, BA; Xu, P; Hall, AK. Wounds increase activin in skin and a vasoactive neuropeptide in sensory ganglia. *Dev. Biol,* 2004 271, 1–10.

Cui, M; Honore, P; Zhong, C; Gauvin, D; Mikusa, J; Hernandez, G; Chandran, P; Gomtsyan, A; Brown, B; Bayburt, EK; Marsh, K; Bianchi, B; McDonald, H; Niforatos, W; Neelands, TR; Moreland, RB; Decker, MW; Lee, CH; Sullivan, JP; Faltynek, CR. TRPV1 receptors in the CNS play a key role in broad-spectrum analgesia of TRPV1 antagonists. *J. Neurosci,* 2006 26, 9385-9393.

Cummins, TR; Aglieco, F; Renganathan, M; Herzog, RI; Dib-Hajj, SD; Waxman, SG. Nav1.3 sodium channels: rapid repriming and slow closed-state inactivation display quantitative differences after expression in a mammalian cell line and in spinal sensory neurons. *J. Neurosci,* 2001 21, 5952–5961.

Cummins, TR; Sheets, PL; Waxman, SG. The roles of sodium channels in nociception: Implications for mechanisms of pain. *Pain,* 2007 131, 243-257.

Cummins, TR; Waxman, SG. Downregulation of tetrodotoxin-resistant sodium currents and upregulation of a rapidly repriming tetrodotoxin-sensitive sodium current in small spinal sensory neurons after nerve injury. *J. Neurosci,* 1997 17, 3503–3514.

Cutrer, FM; Huerter, K. Migraine aura. *Neurologist,* 2007 13, 118-125.

D'Arco, M; Giniatullin, R; Simonetti, M; Fabbro, A; Nair, A; Nistri, A; Fabbretti, E. Neutralization of nerve growth factor induces plasticity of ATP-sensitive P2X3 receptors of nociceptive trigeminal ganglion neurons. *J. Neurosci,* 2007 27, 8190-8201.

Dawbarn, D; Fahey, M; Watson, J; Tyler, S; Shoemark, D; Sessions, R; Zhang, R; Brady, L; Willis, C; Allen, SJ. NGF receptor TrkAd5: therapeutic agent and drug design target. *Biochem. Soc. Trans,* 2006 34, 587-590.

Debeir, T; Saragovi, HU; Cuello, AC. A nerve growth factor mimetic TrkA antagonist causes withdrawal of cortical cholinergic boutons in the adult rat. *Proc. Natl. Acad. Sci. U. S. A,* 1999 96, 4067-4072.

DeLeo, JA; Yezierski, RP. The role of neuroinflammation and neuroimmune activation in persistent pain. *Pain,* 2001 90, 1-6.

Della Seta, D; de Acetis, L; Aloe, L; Alleva, E. NGF effects on hot plate behaviors in mice. *Pharmacol. Biochem. Behav,* 1994 49, 701–705.

Diamond, J; Foerster, A; Holmes, M; Coughlin, M. Sensory nerves in adult rats regenerate and restore sensory function to the skin independently of endogenous NGF. *J. Neurosci*, 1992 12, 1467-1476.

Diener, HC; May, A. New aspects of migraine pathophysiology: lessons learned from positron emission tomography. *Curr. Opin. Neurol,* 1996 9, 199-201.

Di Marco, E; Mathor, M; Bondanza, S; Cutuli, N; Marchisio, PC; Cancedda, R; De Luca M. Nerve growth factor binds to normal human keratinocytes through high and low affinity receptors and stimulates their growth by a novel autocrine loop. *J. Biol. Chem,* 1993 268, 22838-22846.

Diogenes, A; Akopian, AN; Hargreaves, KM. NGF up-regulates TRPA1: implications for orofacial pain. *J. Dent. Res,* 2007 86, 550-555.

Djouhri, L; Dawbarn, D; Robertson, A; Newton, R; Lawson, SN. Time course and nerve growth factor dependence of inflammation-induced alterations in electrophysiological membrane properties in nociceptive primaryafferent neurons. *Neurosci,* 2001 21, 8722-8733.

Dodick, D; Silberstein, S. Central sensitization theory of migraine: clinical implications *Headache,* 2006 46, S182-S191.

Donnelly-Roberts, D; McGaraughty, S; Shieh, CC; Honore, P; Jarvis, MF. Painful purinergic receptors. *J. Pharmacol. Exp. Ther,* 2008 324, 409-415.

Donnerer, J; Liebmann, I; Schicho, R. ERK and STAT3 phosphorylation in sensory neurons during capsaicin –induced impairment and nerve growth factor treatment. *Pharmacology,* 2005 75, 116-121.

Fabbretti, E; D'Arco, M; Fabbro, A; Simonetti, M; Nistri, A; Giniatullin, R. Delayed upregulation of ATP P2X3 receptors of trigeminal sensory neurons by calcitonin gene-related peptide. *J. Neurosci,* 2006 26, 6163-6171.

Facer, P; Casula, MA; Smith, GD; Benham, CD; Chessell, IP; Bountra, C; Sinisi, M; Birch, R; Anand, P. Differential expression of the capsaicin receptor TRPV1 and related novel receptors TRPV3, TRPV4 and TRPM8 in normal human tissues and changes in traumatic and diabetic neuropathy. *BMC Neurol,* 2007 7, 11.

Fitzgerald, M; Wall, PD; Goedert, M; Emson, PC. Nerve growth factor counteracts the neurophysiological and neurochemical effects of chronic sciatic nerve section. *Brain Res,* 1985 332, 131-41.

Fjell, J; Cummins, TR; Fried, K; Black, JA; Waxman, SG. In vivo NGF deprivation reduces SNS expression and TTX-R sodium currents in IB4-negative DRG neurons. *J. Neurophysiol,* 1999 81, 803-810.

Garcia-Larrea, L; Magnin, M. Pathophysiology of neuropathic pain: review of experimental models and proposed mechanisms. *Presse Med,* 2008 37, 315-340.

Gardiner, NJ; Fernyhough, P; Tomlinson, DR; Mayer, U; von der Mark, H; Streuli, CH. Alpha7 integrin mediates neurite outgrowth of distinct populations of adult sensory neurons. *Mol. Cell Neurosci,* 2005 28, 229-240.

Garofalo, L; Ribeiro-da-Silva, A; Cuello, AC. Nerve growth factor-induced synaptogenesis and hypertrophy of cortical cholinergic terminals. *Proc. Natl. Acad. Sci. U. S. A,* 1992 89, 2639-2643.

Giovengo, SL; Russell, IJ; Larson, AA. Increased concentrations of nerve growth factor in cerebrospinal fluid of patients with fibromyalgia. *J. Rheumatol,* 1999 26, 1564-1569.

Gould, HJ 3rd; Gould, TN; England, JD; Paul, D; Liu, ZP; Levinson, SR. A possible role for nerve growth factor in the augmentation of sodium channels in models of chronic pain. *Brain Res,* 2000 854, 19-29.

Govrin-Lippmann, R; Devor, M. Ongoing activity in severed nerves: Source and variation with time. *Brain Res,* 1978 159, 406–410.

Gwak, YS; Nam, TS; Paik, KS; Hulsebosch, CE; Leem, JW. Attenuation of mechanical hyperalgesia following spinal cord injury by administration of antibodies to nerve growth factor in the rat. *Neurosci. Lett,* 2003 336, 117-120.

Halvorson, KG; Kubota, K; Sevcik, MA; Lindsay, TH; Sotillo, JE; Ghilardi, JR; Rosol, TJ; Boustany, L; Shelton, DL; Mantyh, PW. A blocking antibody to nerve growth factor attenuates skeletal pain induced by prostate tumor cells growing in bone. *Cancer Res,* 2005 65, 9426-9435.

Hao, J; Ebendal, T; Xu, X; Wiesenfeld–Hallin, Z; Eriksdottter Jonhagen, M. Intracerebroventricular infusion of nerve growth factor induces pain-like response in rats. *Neurosci. Lett,* 2000 286, 208-212.

Hathway, GJ; Fitzgerald, M. Time course and dose-dependence of nerve growth factor-induced secondary hyperalgesia in the mouse. *J. Pain,* 2006 7, 57-61.

Headache Classification Subcommittee of the International Headache Society. The International Classification of Headache Disorders: 2nd edition. *Cephalalgia,* 2004 24, 9-160.

Hefti, FF; Rosenthal, A; Walicke, PA; Wyatt, S; Vergara, G; Shelton, DL; Davies, AM. Novel class of pain drugs based on antagonism of NGF. *Trends Pharmacol. Sci,* 2006 27, 85-91.

Helyes, Z; Elekes, K; Németh, J; Pozsgai, G; Sándor, K; Kereskai, L; Börzsei, R; Pintér, E; Szabó, A; Szolcsányi, J. Role of transient receptor potential vanilloid 1 receptors in endotoxin-induced airway inflammation in the mouse. *Am. J. Physiol. Lung Cell Mol. Physiol,* 2007 292, L1173-L1181.

Hoheisel, U; Kaske, A; Mense, S. Relationship between neuronal activity and substance P-immunoreactivity in the rat spinal cord during acute and persistent myositis. *Neurosci. Lett,* 1998 257, 21–24.

Huang, J; Zhang, X; McNaughton, PA. Inflammatory pain: the cellular basis of heat hyperalgesia. *Curr. Neuropharmacol.* 2006 4:197-206.

Hulsebosch, CE; Coggeshall, RE. Intraspinal sprouting after administration of nerve growth factor antibodies to neonatal rats. *Brain Res,* 1988 461, 322-327.

Ichikawa H; Yabuuchi T; Jin HW; Terayama, R; Yamaai, T; Deguchi, T; Kamioka, H; Takano-Yamamoto, T; Sugimoto, T. Brain-derived neurotrophic factor-immunoreactive primary sensory neurons in the rat trigeminal ganglion and trigeminal sensory nuclei. *Brain Res,* 2006 1081, 113-118.

Jacobsen, S; Wildschiodtz, G; Danneskiold-Samsoe, B. Isokinetic and isometric muscle strength combined with transcutaneous electrical muscle stimulation in primary fibromyalgia syndrome. *J. Rheumatol,* 1991 18, 1390–1393.

Jarvis, CR; Xiong, ZG; Plant, JR; Churchill, D; Lu, WY; MacVicar, BA; MacDonald, JF. NT modulation of NMDA receptors in cultured murine and isolated rat neurons. *J. Neurophysiol,* 1997 78, 2363-2371.

Jimenez-Andrade, JM; Martin, CD; Koewler, NJ; Freeman, KT; Sullivan, LJ; Halvorson, KG; Barthold, CM; Peters, CM; Buus, RJ; Ghilardi, JR; Lewis, JL; Kuskowski, MA; Mantyh, PW. Nerve growth factor sequestering therapy attenuates non-malignant skeletal pain following fracture. *Pain,* 2007 133, 183-196.

Kalyan-Raman, U; Kalyan-Raman, K; Yunus, M; Masi, A. Muscle pathology in primary fibromyalgia syndrome: a light microscopic, histochemical and ultrastructural study. *J. Rheumatol,* 1984 11, 808–813.

Kanaan, SA; Poole, S; Saade, NE; Jabbur, S; Safieh-Garabedian, B. Interleukin-10 reduces the endotoxin-induced hyperalgesia in mice. *J. Neuroimmunol,* 1998 86, 142–150.

Kassel, O; de Blay, F; Duvernelle, C; Olgart, C; Israel-Biet, D; Krieger, P; Moreau, L; Muller, C; Pauli, G; Frossard, N. Local increase in the number of mast cells and expression of nerve growth factor in the bronchus of asthmatic patients after repeated inhalation of allergen at low-dose. *Clin. Exp. Allergy,* 2001 31, 1432-1440.

Katsura, H; Obata, K; Mizushima, T; Yamanaka, H; Kobayashi, K; Dai, Y; Fukuoka, T; Tokunaga, A; Sakagami, M; Noguchi, K. Antisense knock down of TRPA1, but not TRPM8, alleviates cold hyperalgesia after spinal nerve ligation in rats. *Exp. Neurol,* 2006 200, 112-123.

Katz, WA; Rothenberg, R. Section 3: The nature of pain: pathophysiology. *J. Clin. Rheumatol,* 2005 11, S11-S15.

Kawamoto, K; Aoki, J; Tanaka, A; Itakura, A; Hosono, H; Arai, H; Kiso, Y; Matsuda, H. Nerve growth factor activates mast cells through the collaborative interaction with lysophosphatidylserine expressed on the membrane surface of activated platelets. *J. Immunol,* 2002 168, 6412-6419.

Kerr, BJ; Bradbury, EJ; Bennett, DL; Trivedi, PM; Dassan, P; French, J; Shelton, DB; McMahon, SB; Thompson, SW. Brain-derived neurotrophic factor modulates nociceptive sensory inputs and NMDA-evoked responses in the rat spinal cord. *J. Neurosci,* 1999 19, 5138-5148.

Kerr, BJ; Souslova, V; McMahon, SB; Wood, JN. A role for the TTX-resistant sodium channel Nav 1.8 in NGF-induced hyperalgesia, but not neuropathic pain. *Neuroreport,* 2001 12, 3077-3080.

Khan, GM; Chen, SR; Pan, HL. Role of primary afferent nerves in allodynia caused by diabetic neuropathy in rats. *Neuroscience,* 2002 114, 291-299.

Khasar, SG; Lia, YH; Martin, A; Dadgar, J; McMahon, T; Wang, D; Hundle, B; Aley, KO; Isemberg, W; McKarter, G; Green, PC; Hodge, CW; Levine

JD; Messing, RO. A novel nociceptor signaling pathway revealed in protein kinase C epsilon mutant mice. *Neuron,* 1999 24, 253-260.

Kitamura, N; Konno, A; Kuwahara, T; Komagiri, Y. Nerve growth factor-induced hyperexcitability of rat sensory neuron in culture. *Biomed. Res,* 2005 26, 123-130.

Koltzenburg, M; Bennett, DL; Shelton, DL; McMahon, SB. Neutralization of endogenous NGF prevents the sensitization of nociceptors supplying inflamed skin. *Eur. J. Neurosci,* 1999 11, 1698-1704.

Krenz, NR; Weaver, LC. Nerve growth factor in glia and inflammatory cells of the injured rat spinal cord. *J. Neurochem,* 2000 74, 730–739.

Larkin, M. Nerve growth factor promising in diabetic neuropathy...and in HIV-1-related neuropathy. *Lancet,* 1998 352, 1039.

Lee, YJ; Zachrisson, O; Tonge, DA; McNaughton, PA. Upregulation of bradykinin B2 receptor expression by neurotrophic factors and nerve injury in mouse sensory neurons. *Mol. Cell Neurosci,* 2002 19, 186-200.

Leffler, A; Cummins, TR; Dib-Hajj, SD; Hormuzdiar, WN; Black, JA; Waxman, SG. GDNF and NGF reverse changes in repriming of TTX-sensitive Na(+) currents following axotomy of dorsal root ganglion neurons. *J. Neurophysiol,* 2002 88, 650-658.

Leon, A; Buriani, A; Dal Toso, R; Fabris, M; Romanello, S; Aloe, L; Levi-Montalcini, R. Mast cells synthesize, store, and release nerve growth factor. *Proc. Natl. Acad. Sci. U. S. A,* 1994 91, 3739-3743.

LeSauteur, L; Wei, L; Gibbs, BF; Saragovi, HU. Small peptide mimics of nerve growth factor bind TrkA receptors and affect biological responses. *J. Biol. Chem,* 1995 270, 6564-6569.

Levi-Montalcini, R; Skaper, SD; Dal Toso, R; Petrelli, L; Leon, A. Nerve growth factor: From neurotrophin to neurokine. *Trends Neurosci,* 1996 19, 514–520.

Levine, JD; Alessandri-Haber, N. TRP channels: targets for the relief of pain. *Biochim. Biophys. Acta,* 2007 1772, 989-1003.

Levy, D; Burstein, R; Strassman, AM. Mast cell involvement in the pathophysiology of migraine headache: A hypothesis. *Headache,* 2006 46, S13-S18.

Lewin, GR; Rueff, A; Mendell, LM. Peripheral and central mechanisms of NGF-induced hyperalgesia. *Eur. J. Neurosci*, 1994 6, 1903-1912.

Lindholm, D; Hengerer, B; Heumann, R; Carroll, P; Thoenen, H. Glucocorticoid hormones negatively regulate nerve growth factor expression in vivo and in cultured rat fibroblasts. *Eur. J. Neurosci,* 1990 2, 795-801.

Lu, VB; Ballanyi, K; Colmers, WF; Smith, PA. Neuron type-specific effects of brain-derived neurotrophic factor in rat superficial dorsal horn and their relevance to 'central sensitization'. *J. Physiol,* 2007 584, 543-563.

Ma, QP; Woolf, CJ. The progressive tactile hyperalgesia induced by peripheral inflammation is nerve growth factor dependent. *Neuroreport,* 1997 8, 807-810.

MacQueen, GM; Ramakrishnan, K; Croll, SD; Siuciak, JA; Yu, G; Young, LT; Fahnestock, M. Performance of heterozygous brain-derived neurotrophic factor knockout mice on behavioral analogues of anxiety, nociception, and depression. *Behav. Neurosci,* 2001 115, 1145-1153.

Malcangio, M; Garrett, NE; Tomlinson, DR. Nerve growth factor treatment increases stimulus-evoked release of sensory neuropeptides in the rat spinal cord. *Eur. J. Neurosci,* 1997 9, 1101-1104.

Malcangio, M; Ramer, MS; Boucher, TJ; McMahon, SB. Intrathecally injected neurotrophins and the release of substance P from the rat isolated spinal cord. *Eur. J .Neurosci,* 2000 12, 139-144.

Malick, A; Burstein, R. Peripheral and central sensitization during migraine. *Funct. Neurol,* 2000 15, 28-35.

Malik-Hall, M; Dina, OA; Levine, JD. Primary afferent nociceptor mechanisms mediating NGF-induced mechanical hyperalgesia. *Eur. J. Neurosci,* 2005 21, 3387-3394.

Mamet, J; Lazdunski, M; Voilley, N. How nerve growth factor drives physiological and inflammatory expressions of acid-sensing ion channel 3 in sensory neurons. *Biol. Chem,* 2003 278, 48907-48913.

Mannion, RJ; Costigan, M; Decosterd, I; Amaya, F; Ma, QP; Holstege, JC; Ji, RR; Acheson, A; Lindsay, RM; Wilkinson, GA; Woolf, CJ. Neurotrophins: peripherally and centrally acting modulators of tactile stimulus-induced inflammatory pain hypersensitivity. *Proc. Natl. Acad. Sci. U. S. A,* 1999 96, 9385-9390.

Marcol, W; Kotulska, K; Larysz-Brysz, M; Kowalik, JL. BDNF contributes to animal model neuropathic pain after peripheral nerve transection. *Neurosurg. Rev,* 2007 30, 235-243.

Matzner, O; Devor, M. Hyperexcitability at sites of nerve injury depends on voltage-sensitive Na^+ channels. *J. Neurophysiol,* 1994 72, 349–359.

May, A; Matharu, M. New insights into migraine: application of functional and structural imaging. *Curr. Opin. Neurol,* 2007 20, 306-309.

McArthur, JC; Yiannoutsos, C; Simpson, DM; Adornato, BT; Singer, EJ; Hollander, H; Marra, C; Rubin, M; Cohen, BA; Tucker, T; Navia, BA; Schifitto, G; Katzenstein, D; Rask, C; Zaborski, L; Smith, ME; Shriver, S;

Millar, L; Clifford, DB; Karalnik, IJ. A phase II trial of nerve growth factor for sensory neuropathy associated with HIV infection. AIDS Clinical Trials Group Team 291. *Neurology,* 2000 54, 1080-1088.

McMahon, SB. NGF as a mediator of inflammatory pain. *Philos. Trans. R. Soc. Lond. B. Biol. Sci,* 1996 351, 431-440.

Mendell, LM; Albers, KM; Davis, BM. Neurotrophins, nociceptors, and pain. *Microsc. Res. Tech,* 1999 45, 252-261.

Meuser, T; Pietruck, C; Gabriel, A; Xie, GX; Lim, KJ; Pierce Palmer, P. 5-HT7 receptors are involved in mediating 5-HT-induced activation of rat primary afferent neurons. *Life Sci,* 2002 71, 2279-2289.

Michael, GJ; Averill, S; Nitkunan, A; Rattray, M; Bennett, DL; Yan, Q; Priestley, JV. Nerve growth factor treatment increases brain-derived neurotrophic factor selectively in TrkA-expressing dorsal root ganglion cells and in their central terminations within the spinal cord. *J. Neurosci,* 1997 17, 8476–8490.

Mizisin, AP; Shelton, GD; Wagner, S; Rusbridge, C; Powell, HC. Myelin splitting, Schwann cell injury and demyelination in feline diabetic neuropathy. *Acta Neuropathol,* 1998 95, 171-174.

Molliver, DC; Lindsay, J; Albers, KM; Davis, BM. Overexpression of NGF or GDNF alters transcriptional plasticity evoked by inflammation. *Pain,* 2005 113, 277-284.

Mousa, SA; Cheppudira, BP; Shaqura, M; Fischer, O; Hofmann, J; Hellweg, R; Schäfer, M. Nerve growth factor governs the enhanced ability of opioids to suppress inflammatory pain. *Brain,* 2007 130, 502-513.

Nicol, GD; Vasko, MR. Unraveling the story of NGF-mediated sensitization of nociceptive sensory neurons: ON or OFF the Trks? *Mol. Interv,* 2007 7, 26-41.

Noguchi, K; Obata, K; Dai, Y. Changes in DRG neurons and spinal excitability in neuropathy. *Novartis Found Symp,* 2004 261, 103-110.

Numazaki, M; Tominaga, M. Nociception and TRP Channels. *Curr Drug Targets CNS Neurol. Disord,* 2004 3, 479-485.

Oaklander, AL. Mechanisms of pain and itch caused by herpes zoster (shingles). *J. Pain,* 2008 9, S10-S18.

Obata, K; Katsura, H; Mizushima, T; Yamanaka, H; Kobayashi, K; Dai, Y; Fukuoka, T; Tokunaga, A; Tominaga, M; Noguchi, K. TRPA1 induced in sensory neurons contributes to cold hyperalgesia after inflammation and nerve injury. *J. Clin. Invest,* 2005 115, 2393-2401.

Obata, K; Yamanaka, H; Dai, Y; Mizushima, T; Fukuoka, T. Contribution of degeneration of motor and sensory fibers to pain behavior and the changes in neurotrophic factors in rat dorsal root ganglion. *Exp. Neurol,* 2004a 188, 149–160.

Obata, K; Yamanaka, H; Dai, Y; Mizushima, T; Fukuoka, T; Tokunaga, A; Noguchi, K. Differential activation of MAPK in injured and uninjured DRG neurons following chronic constriction injury of the sciatic nerve in rats. *Eur. J. Neurosci,* 2004b 20, 2881-2895.

Okuse, K; Chaplan, SR; McMahon, SB; Luo, ZD; Calcutt, NA; Scott, BP; Akopian, AN; Wood, JN. Regulation of expression of the sensory neuron-specific sodium channel SNS in inflammatory and neuropathic pain. *Mol. Cell Neurosci,* 1997 10, 196-207.

Omoigui, S. The biochemical origin of pain: the origin of all pain is inflammation and the inflammatory response, Part 2 of 3 – inflammatory profile of pain syndromes. *Med. Hypotheses*, 2007 69, 1169-1178.

Owolabi, JB; Rizkalla, G; Tehim, A; Ross, GM; Riopelle, RJ; Kamboj, R; Ossipov, M; Bian, D; Wegert, S; Porreca, F; Lee, DK. Characterization of antiallodynic actions of ALE-0540, a novel nerve growth factor receptor antagonist, in the rat. *J. Pharmacol. Exp. Ther,* 1999 289, 1271-1276.

Padilla, F; Couble, ML; Coste, B; Maingret, F; Clerc, N; Crest, M; Ritter, AM; Magloire, H; Delmas, P. Expression and localization of the Nav1.9 sodium channel in enteric neurons and in trigeminal sensory endings: implication for intestinal reflex function and orofacial pain. *Mo. Cell Neurosci,* 2007 35, 138-152.

Palazzo, E; Rossi, F; Maione, S. Role of TRPV1 receptors in descending modulation of pain. *Mol. Cell Endocrinol,* 2008 286, S79-S83.

Park, SY; Choi, JY; Kim, RU; Lee, YS; Cho, HJ; Kim, DS. Downregulation of voltage-gated potassium channel alpha gene expression by axotomy and neurotrophins in rat dorsal root ganglia. *Mol. Cells,* 2003 16, 256-259.

Petersen, KL; Rowbotham, MC. Will ion-channel blockers be useful for management of nonneuropathic pain? *J. Pain,* 2000 1, 26-34.

Petrenko, AB; Yamakura, T; Baba, H; Shimoji, K. The role of N-methyl-D-aspartate (NMDA) receptors in pain: a review. *Anesth. Analg,* 2003 97, 1108-1116.

Petzke, F; Clauw, DJ; Ambrose, K; Khine, A; Gracely, RH. Increased pain sensitivity in fibromyalgia: effects of stimulus type and mode of presentation. *Pain,* 2003 105, 403-413.

Pezet, S; McMahon, SB. NTs: Mediators and modulators of pain. *Annu. Rev. Neurosci,* 2006 29, 507–538.

Pezet, S; Cunningham, J; Patel, J; Grist, J; Gavazzi, I; Lever, IJ; Malcangio, M. BDNF modulates sensory neuron synaptic activity by a facilitation of

GABA transmission in the dorsal horn. *Mol. Cell Neurosci,* 2002 21, 51-62.

Pezet, S; Onténiente, B; Grannec, G; Calvino, B. Chronic pain is associated with increased TrkA immunoreactivity in spinoreticular neurons. *Neurosci,* 1999 19, 5482-5492.

Price, DD; Staud, R; Robinson, ME; Mauderli, AP; Cannon, R; Vierck, CJ. Enhanced temporal summation of second pain and its central modulation in fibromyalgia patients. *Pain,* 2002 99, 49-59.

Price, DD; Staud, R. Neurobiology of fibromyalgia syndrome. *J. Rheumatol. Suppl,* 2005 75, 22-28.

Price, TJ; Louria, MD; Candelario-Soto, D; Dussor, GO; Jeske, NA; Patwardhan, AM; Diogenes, A; Trott, AA; Hargreaves, KM; Flores, CM. Treatment of trigeminal ganglion neurons in vitro with NGF, GDNF or BDNF: effects on neuronal survival, neurochemical properties and TRPV1-mediated neuropeptide secretion. *BMC Neurosci,* 2005 6, 4.

Quintão, NL; Santos, AR; Campos, MM; Calixto, JB. The role of neurotrophic factors in genesis and maintenance of mechanical hypernociception after brachial plexus avulsion in mice. *Pain,* 2008 136, 125-133.

Ramer, MS; French, GD; Bisby, MA. Wallerian degeneration is required for both neuropathic pain and sympathetic sprouting into the DRG. *Pain,* 1997 72, 71-78.

Ramer, MS; Kawaja, MD; Henderson, JT; Roder, JC; Bisby, MA. Glial overexpression of NGF enhances neuropathic pain and adrenergic sprouting into DRG following chronic sciatic constriction in mice. *Neurosci. Lett,* 1998 251, 53-56.

Ramer, MS; Bradbury, EJ; McMahon, SB. Nerve growth factor induces P2X(3) expression in sensory neurons. *J. Neurochem,* 2001 77, 864-875.

Reuter, U; Bolay, H; Jansen-Olesen, I; Chiarugi, A; Sanchez del Rio, M; Letourneau, R; Theoharides, TC; Waeber, C; Moskowitz, MA. Delayed inflammation in rat meninges: implications for migraine pathophysiology. *Brain,* 2001 124, 2490-2502.

Reuter, U; Chiarugi, A; Bolay, H; Moskowitz, MA. Nuclear factor-kappaB as a molecular target for migraine therapy. *Ann. Neurol,* 2002 51, 507-516.

Ritter, AM; Lewin, GR; Kremer, NE; Mendell, LM. Requirement for nerve growth factor in the development of myelinated nociceptors in vivo. *Nature,* 1991 350, 500–502.

Ro, LS; Chang, KH. Neuropathic pain: mechanisms and treatments. *Chang Gung Med. J,* 2005 28, 597-605.

Ro, LS; Chen, ST; Tang, LM; Jacobs, JM. Effect of NGF and anti-NGF on neuropathic pain in rats following chronic constriction injury of the sciatic nerve. *Pain,* 1999 79, 265-274.

Roberts, LA; Connor, M. TRPV1 antagonists as a potential treatment for hyperalgesia. *Recent Patents CNS Drug Discov,* 2006 1, 65-76.

Romero, MI; Rangappa, N; Garry, MG; Smith, GM. Functional regeneration of chronically injured sensory afferents into adult spinal cord after neurotrophin gene therapy. *Neurosci,* 2001 21, 8408-8416.

Ruiz, G; Baños, JE. The effect of endoneurial nerve growth factor on calcitonin gene-related peptide expression in primary sensory neurons. *Brain Res,* 2005 1042, 44-52.

Saban, MR; Nguyen, NB; Hammond, TG; Saban, R. Gene expression profiling of mouse bladder inflammatory responses to LPS, substance P, and antigen-stimulation. *Am. J. Pathol,* 2002 160, 2095–2110.

Sabsovich, I; Wei, T; Guo, TZ; Zhao, R; Shi, X; Li, X; Yeomans, DC; Klyukinov, M; Kingery, WS; Clark, JD. Effect of anti-NGF antibodies in a rat tibia fracture model of complex regional pain syndrome type I. *Pain,* 2008 138, 47-60.

Safieh-Garabedian, B; Dardenne, M; Pleau, JM; Saade, NE. Potent analgesic and anti-inflammatory actions of a novel thymulin-related peptide in the rat. *Br. J. Pharmacol,* 2002 136, 947–955.

Salter, MW. Cellular signalling pathways of spinal pain neuroplasticity as targets for analgesic development. *Curr Top Med Chem,* 2005 5, 557-567.

Sanchez-Del-Rio, M; Reuter, U; Moskowitz, MA. New insights into migraine pathophysiology. *Curr. Opin. Neurol,* 2006 19, 294-298.

Saragovi, HU; Gehring, K. Development of pharmacological agents for targeting NTs and their receptors. *Trends Pharmacol. Sci,* 2000 21, 93-98.

Sarchielli, P; Alberti, A; Baldi, A; Coppola, F; Rossi, C; Pierguidi, L; Floridi, A; Calabresi, P. Proinflammatory cytokines, adhesion molecules, and lymphocyte integrin expression in the internal jugular blood of migraine patients without aura assessed ictally. *Headache,* 2006a 46, 200-207.

Sarchielli, P; Alberti, A; Coppola, F; Baldi, A; Gallai, B; Floridi, A; Floridi, A; Capocchi, G; Gallai, V. Platelet-activating factor (PAF) in internal jugular venous blood of migraine without aura patients assessed during migraine attacks. *Cephalalgia,* 2004b 24, 623-630.

Sarchielli, P; Alberti, A; Floridi, A; Gallai, V. Levels of nerve growth factor in cerebrospinal fluid of chronic daily headache patients. *Neurology,* 2001 57, 132-134.

Sarchielli, P; Alberti, A; Gallai, B; Coppola, F; Baldi, A; Floridi, A; Gallai, V. Brain-derived neurotrophic factor in cerebrospinal fluid of patients with chronic daily headache: relationship with nerve growth factor and glutamate levels. *J. Headache Pain,* 2002 3, 129-135.

Sarchielli, P; Di Filippo, M; Nardi, K; Calabresi, P. Sensitization, glutamate, and the link between migraine and fibromyalgia. *Curr. Pain Headache Rep,* 2007a 11, 343-351.

Sarchielli, P; Mancini, ML; Floridi, A; Coppola, F; Rossi, C; Nardi, K; Acciarresi, M; Pini, LA; Calabresi, P. Increased levels of neurotrophins are not specific for chronic migraine: evidence from primary fibromyalgia syndrome. *J. Pain,* 2007b 8, 737-745.

Sarchielli, P; Floridi, A; Mancini, ML; Rossi, C; Coppola, F; Baldi, A; Pini, LA; Calabresi, P. NF-kappaB activity and iNOS expression in monocytes from internal Jugular blood of migraine without aura patients during attacks. *Cephalalgia,* 2006b 26, 1071-1079.

Sarchielli, P; Gallai, V. Nerve growth factor and chronic daily headache: a potential implication for therapy. *Expert Rev. Neurother,* 2004a 4, 115-127.

Schifitto, G; Yiannoutsos, C; Simpson, DM; Adornato, BT; Singer, EJ; Hollander, H; Marra, CM; Rubin, M; Cohen, BA; Tucker, T; Koralnik, IJ; Katzenstein, D; Haidich, B; Smith, ME; Shriver, S; Millar, L; Clifford, DB; McArthur, JC; AIDS Clinical Trials Group Team 291. Long-term treatment with recombinant nerve growth factor for HIV-associated sensory neuropathy. *Neurology,* 2001 57, 1313-1316.

Scholz, J; Woolf, CJ. Can we conquer pain? *Nat. Neurosci,* 2002 5, 1062–1067.

Schwartz, F; Brodie, C; Appel, E; Kazimirsky, G; Shainberg, A. Effect of helium/neon laser irradiation on nerve growth factor synthesis and secretion in skeletal muscle cultures. *Photochem. Photobiol B,* 2002 66, 195-200.

Sevcik, MA; Ghilardi, JR; Peters, CM; Lindsay, TH; Halvorson, KG; Jonas, BM; Kubota, K; Kuskowski, MA; Boustany, L; Shelton, DL; Mantyh, PW. Anti-NGF therapy profoundly reduces bone cancer pain and the accompanying increase in markers of peripheral and central sensitization. *Pain,* 2005 115, 128-141.

Shu, XQ; Mendell, LM. Neurotrophins and hyperalgesia. *Proc. Natl. Acad. Sci. U. S. A.* 1999 96, 7693-7696.

Siddall, PJ; Cousins, MJ. Spinal pain mechanisms. *Spine,* 1997 22, 98–104.

Silberstein, SD. Migraine pathophysiology and its clinical implications *Cephalalgia,* 2004 24, 2-7.

Simonetti, M; Fabbro, A; D'Arco, M; Zweyer, M; Nistri, A; Giniatullin, R; Fabbretti, E. Comparison of P2X and TRPV1 receptors in ganglia or primary culture of trigeminal neurons and their modulation by NGF or serotonin. *Mol. Pain,* 2006 2, 11.

Skaper, SD; Pollock, M; Facci, L. Mast cells differentially express and release active high molecular weight neurotrophins. *Brain Res. Mol. Brain Res,* 2001 97, 177-185.

Soderling, TR; Derkach, VA. Postsynaptic protein phosphorylation and LTP. *Trends Neurosci,* 2000 23, 75-80.

Sorensen, J; Graven-Nielsen, T; Henriksson, KG; Bengtsson, M; Arendt-Nielsen, L. Hyperexcitability in fibromyalgia. *J. Rheumatol,* 1998 25, 152-155.

Spiegel, K; Agrafiotis, D; Caprathe, B; Davis, RE; Dickerson, MR; Fergus, JH; Hepburn, TW; Marks, JS; Van Dorf, M; Wieland, DM; et al. PD 90780, a non peptide inhibitor of nerve growth factor's binding to the P75 NGF receptor. *Biochem. Biophys. Res. Commun,* 1995 217, 488-494.

Staud, R; Cannon, RC; Mauderli, AP; Robinson, ME; Price, DD; Vierck, CJ. Temporal summation of pain from mechanical stimulation of muscle tissue in normal controls and subjects with fibromyalgia syndrome. *Pain,* 2003 102, 87-95.

Staud, R; Price, DD; Robinson, ME; Mauderli, AP; Vierck, CJ. Maintenance of windup of second pain requires less frequent stimulation in fibromyalgia patients compared to normal controls. *Pain,* 2004 110, 689-696.

Staud, R; Rodriguez, ME. Mechanisms of disease: pain in fibromyalgia syndrome. *Nat. Clin. Pract. Rheumatol,* 2006 2, 90-98.

Staud, R; Vierck, CJ; Cannon, RL; Mauderli, AP; Price, DD. Abnormal sensitization and temporal summation of second pain (wind-up) in patients with fibromyalgia syndrome. *Pain,* 2001 91, 165–175.

Steiner, P; Pfeilschifter, J; Boeckh, C; Radeke, H; Otten, U. Interleukin-1 beta and tumor necrosis factor-alpha synergistically stimulate nerve growth factor synthesis in rat mesangial cells. *Am. J. Physiol,* 1991 261, F792-F798.

Sugiyama, K; Suzuki, Y; Furuta, H. Histamine-release induced by 7S nerve-growth factor of mouse submandibular salivary glands. *Arch. Oral Biol.* 1985 30, 93-95.

Summer, GJ; Puntillo, KA; Miaskowski, C; Dina, OA; Green, PG; Levine, JD. TrkA and PKC-epsilon in thermal burn-induced mechanical hyperalgesia in the rat. *J. Pain,* 2006 7, 884-891.

Sutherland, SP; Cook, SP; McCleskey, EW. Chemical mediators of pain due to tissue damage and ischemia. *Prog. Brain Res,* 2000 129, 21-38.

Svensson, P; Cairns, BE; Wang, K; Arendt-Nielsen, L. Injection of nerve growth factor into human masseter muscle evokes long-lasting mechanical allodynia and hyperalgesia. *Pain,* 2003 104, 241–247.

Talhouk, RS; Saade, NE; Mouneimne, G; Masaad, CA; Safieh-Garabedian, B. Growth hormone releasing hormone reverses endotoxon-induced localized inflammatory hyperalgesia without reducing the upregulated cytokines, nerve growth factor and gelatinase activity. *Prog. Neuropsychopharmacol. Biol. Psychiatry,* 2004 28, 625-631.

Toma, H; Winston, J; Micci, MA; Shenoy, M; Pasricha, PJ. Nerve growth factor expression is up-regulated in the rat model of L-arginine-induced acute pancreatitis. *Gastroenterology,* 2000 119, 1373-1381.

Torcia, M; Bracci-Laudiero, L; Lucibello, M; Nencioni, L; Labardi, D; Rubartelli, A; Cozzolino, F; Aloe, L; Garaci, E. Nerve growth factor is an autocrine survival factor for memory B lymphocytes. *Cell,* 1996 85, 345-356.

Ueda, M; Hirose, M; Takei, N; Ibuki, T; Naruse, Y; Amaya, F; Ibata, Y; Tanaka, M. Nerve growth factor induces systemic hyperalgesia after thoracic burn injury in the rat. *Neurosci. Lett,* 2002 328, 97–100.

Ueyama, T; Hamada, M; Hano, T; Nishio, I; Masuyama, Y; Furukawa, S. Production of nerve growth factor by cultured vascular smooth muscle cells from spontaneously hypertensive and Wistar-Kyoto rats. *J. Hypertens,* 1993 11, 1061-1065.

Ugolini, G; Marinelli, S; Covaceuszach, S; Cattaneo, A; Pavone, F. The function neutralizing anti-TrkA antibody MNAC13 reduces inflammatory and neuropathic pain. *PNAS,* 2007 104, 2985-2990.

Vedder, H; Affolter, HU; Otten, U. Nerve growth factor (NGF) regulates tachykinin gene expression and biosynthesis in rat sensory neurons during early postnatal development. *Neuropeptides,* 1993 24, 351-357.

Verge, VM; Merlio, JP; Grondin, J; Ernfors, P; Persson, H; Riopelle, RJ; Hökfelt, T; Richardson, PM. Colocalization of NGF binding sites, trk mRNA, and low-affinity NGF receptor mRNA in primary sensory neurons: responses to injury and infusion of NGF. *J. Neurosci,* 1992 12, 4011-4022.

Vikelis, M; Mitsikostas, DD. The role of glutamate and its receptors in migraine. *CNS Neurol. Disord. Drug Targets,* 2007 6, 251-257.

Wall, PD; Gutnick, M. Ongoing activity in peripheral nerves: The physiology and pharmacology of impulses originating from a neuroma. *Exp. Neurol,* 1974 43, 580–593.

Wallace, D; Kinker-Israeli, M; Hallegua, D; Silverman, S; Silver, DM. Cytokines play an aetiopathogenetic role in fibromyalgia: a hypothesis and pilot study. *Rheumatology,* 2001 40, 743–749.

Wan, L; Luo, A; Yu, H; Tian, Y. Effect of touch-stimulus on the expression of C-fos and TrkA in spinal cord following chronic constriction injury of the sciatic nerve in rats. *J. Huazhong Univ. Sci. Technolog. Med. Sci,* 2005 25, 219-222.

Wanigasekara, Y; Keast, JR. Nerve growth factor, glial cell line-derived neurotrophic factor and neurturin prevent semaphorin 3A-mediated growth cone collapse in adult sensory neurons. *Neuroscience,* 2006 142, 369-379.

Wehrman, T; He, X; Raab, B; Dukipatti, A; Blau, H; Garcia, KC. Structural and mechanistic insights into nerve growth factor interactions with the TrkA and p75 receptors. *Neuron,* 2007 53, 25-38.

Weis, J; Dimpfel, W; Schröder, JM. Nerve conduction changes and fine structural alterations of extra- and intrafusal muscle and nerve fibers in streptozotocin diabetic rats. *Muscle Nerve,* 1995 8, 175-184.

Wiesmann, C; de Vos, AM. Nerve growth factor: structure and function. *Cell Mol. Life Sci,* 2001 58, 748-759.

Wild, KD; Bian, D; Zhu, D; Davis, J; Bannon, AW; Zhang, TJ; Louis, JC. Antibodies to nerve growth factor reverse established tactile allodynia in rodent models of neuropathic pain without tolerance. *J. Pharmacol. Exp. Ther,* 2007 322, 282-287.

Wilson-Gerwing, TD; Verge, VM. Neurotrophin-3 attenuates galanin expression in the chronic constriction injury model of neuropathic pain. *Neuroscience,* 2006 141, 2075-2085.

Wolfe, F; Smythe, HA; Yunus, MB; Bennett, RM; Bombardier, C; Goldenberg, DL; Tugwell, P; Campbell, SM; Abeles, M; Clark, P; et al. The American College of Rheumatology 1990 Criteria for the Classification of Fibromyalgia. Report of the Multicenter Criteria Committee. *Arthritis Rheum,* 1990 33, 160–172.

Woodall, AJ; Richards, MA; Turner, DJ; Fitzgerald, EM. Growth factors differentially regulate neuronal Ca(v) channels via ERK-dependent signalling. *Cell Calcium,* 2008 43, 562-575.

Woolf, CJ; Allchorne, A; Safieh-Garabedian, B; Poole, S. Cytokines, nerve growth factor and inflammatory hyperalgesia: the contribution of tumour necrosis factor alpha. *J. Pharmacol,* 1997 121, 417-424.

Woolf, CJ; Chong, MS. Preemptive analgesia: Treating postoperative pain by preventing the establishment of central sensitization. *Anesth. Analg,* 1993 77, 362–379.

Woolf, CJ; Ma, QP; Allchorne, A; Poole, S. Peripheral cell types contributing to the hyperalgesic action of nerve growth factor in inflammation. *J. Neurosci,* 1996 16, 2716-2723.

Wu, C; Boustany, L; Liang, H; Brennan, TJ. Nerve growth factor expression after plantar incision in the rat. *Anesthesiology,* 2007 107, 128-135.

Xu, P; Hall, AK. Activin acts with nerve growth factor to regulate calcitonin gene-related peptide mRNA in sensory neurons. *Neuroscience,* 2007 150, 665-674.

Xue, Q; Jong, B; Chen, T; Schumacher, MA. Transcription of rat TRPV1 utilizes a dual promoter system that is positively regulated by nerve growth factor. *Neurochem,* 2007 101, 212-222.

Yajima, Y; Narita, M; Narita, M; Matsumoto, N; Suzuki, T. Involvement of a spinal brain-derived neurotrophic factor/full-length TrkB pathway in the development of nerve injury-induced thermal hyperalgesia in mice. *Brain Res.* 2002 958, 338-346.

Yajima, Y; Narita, M; Usui, A; Kaneko, C; Miyatake, M; Narita, M; Yamaguchi, T; Tamaki, H; Wachi, H; Seyama, Y; Suzuki, T. Direct evidence for the involvement of brain-derived neurotrophic factor in the development of a neuropathic pain-like state in mice. *J. Neurochem.* 2005 93, 584-594.

Zahn, PK; Subieta, A; Park, SS; Brennan, TJ. Effect of blockade of nerve growth factor and tumor necrosis factor on pain behaviors after plantar incision. *J. Pain,* 2004 5, 157–163.

Zhang, X; Huang, J; McNaughton, PA. NGF rapidly increases membrane expression of TRPV1 heat-gated ion channels. *EMBO J,* 2005 24, 4211-4223.

Zhu, W; Oxford, GS. Phosphoinositide-3-kinase and mitogen activated protein kinase signaling pathways mediate acute NGF sensitization of TRPV1. *Mol. Cell Neurosci,* 2007 34, 689-700.

Zhuang, ZY; Xu, H; Clapham, DE; Ji, RR. Phosphatidylinositol 3-kinase activates ERK in primary sensory neurons and mediates inflammatory heat hyperalgesia through TRPV1 sensitization. *J. Neurosci,* 2004 24, 8300-8309.

INDEX

A

H

I

N

O

P